Contents

Foreword

In the 1990s nurses were given prescribing rights using a rather limited formulary. This role has been evaluated positively and recently their prescribing rights have been expanded. These are set to expand further in the future and other disciplines such as the allied health professions will be provided with prescribing privileges. However, on reading *How Drugs Work* I realised that this book should also be required reading for mid-career doctors, pharmacists and dentists who wish to update their knowledge on pharmacology. Therefore, the first thing to note about this book is that all members of the multiprofessional healthcare team will find it a useful resource.

Pharmacology textbooks are usually written by pharmacologists and it is intriguing to see a book entering the marketplace that is written by a general practitioner. General practitioners understand prescribing better than most. Hugh McGavock is no different but he also possesses in-depth knowledge of the science of pharmacology. Before I first met Hugh I had become aware through comments made by students and colleagues that he was an expert in the field of pharmacology and therapeutics. While this is not in itself unique, I was also made aware that he had a knack of sharing this knowledge with others. He can make the complex simple and the wearisome fascinating. These are gifts that all teachers crave.

The stimulus for this book has been the excellent feedback that Hugh has received from students and fellow teachers. Many have urged him to put his unique knowledge and expertise down on paper. However, there is always a risk that good teaching materials do not transfer well into a good textbook. In *How Drugs Work: basic pharmacology for healthcare professionals,* nothing has been lost in the transition. What we have is a user friendly but rigorous presentation of basic pharmacology. The easy style and 'readability' of the book is one of its most pleasing features and the artwork, information boxes and key points give structure to the book, as well as helping to engage its readers. Its slim volume will be acceptable to many health professionals who are turned off by the normal heavy tomes on the subject. The short chapters are interesting and authoritative and can be read on a 'stand alone' basis, allowing readers to 'dip in and out'.

This book has arrived at an opportune time. Healthcare professionals are extending their prescribing role and it is felt that this will have positive effects on patient care. However, to prescribe without knowing basic pharmacology would be like starting a new journey without a map. This book is one of the best maps of the pharmacology terrain that I have come across.

Professor Hugh McKenna
Head of School of Health Sciences
University of Ulster
October 2002

Preface

The science of medicinal chemicals – pharmacology – is vast and very new, most of it emerging over the past four decades. Consequently, the average student textbook of pharmacology is now around 700 pages long, making it unsuitable for students taking short vocational courses requiring just enough pharmacology to make them informed, safe and effective prescribers, for example, as prescribing nurse practitioners. Such long textbooks are equally unsuitable for doctors, pharmacists and dentists in mid-career, who wish to update their knowledge.

This book sets itself the target of condensing only those aspects of pharmacology of direct relevance to everyday prescribing, into a volume of under 150 pages, without sacrificing accuracy. The intention has been to provide a clear and interesting description of the modern understanding of drug absorption, distribution, action, metabolism, excretion, and adverse effects, equipping readers with a set of clear concepts on which to base their future prescribing decisions. Medical and pharmacy students, too, may benefit from this book as an introduction to the more detailed texts.

Twelve of the chapters were originally published by the GP journal, *Prescriber*, as a series on basic pharmacology. I am greatly indebted to Tim Dean and Emma Handley of *Prescriber*, to their scientific art department, to Professor Tom Walley of Liverpool University (who, with Professor Tony Avery of Nottingham University, refereed the series), and to Beverley McMaster, for her secretarial support. I would also like to thank the staff at Radcliffe Medical Press.

Readers should note that this book describes how drugs work. It is not a textbook of therapeutics (the choice of specific drugs to treat specific diseases), but it contains the science upon which therapeutics (good prescribing) is based. Quality prescribing is an applied science, matching the pharmacology to the diagnosis. Every prescription is an experiment; and powerful modern drugs require scientific understanding if their benefits are to be realised and their many risks minimised.

Hugh McGavock
Cloughmills, Co. Antrim
October 2002

To my dear wife, Betty, and sons, James, Sam and Philip.

1 Getting a drug into the body: absorption

It may seem a truism to state that unless a drug is absorbed into the body in sufficient amounts, it will not work.

However, prescribers are often unaware that the drug industry spends perhaps a quarter of its research budget for a new drug on pharmaceutics, i.e. devising the right presentation to ensure that the drug is effectively absorbed, properly distributed, and remains at its site of action long enough to produce an effect. This is often a major problem whose solution we clinicians take for granted, but it may have involved intense research activity and many millions of pounds of research investment.

Of course, this process is by no means a recent development. Over the past 40 years, the following advances have been made:

- capsules and enteric coatings (EC), which avoid, for example, degradation by gastric acid
- modified-release (MR) tablets, which extend the duration of action
- prodrugs, which use the body's metabolic processes to convert agents into an active compound
- patches for transdermal drug delivery
- dermal implants for long-term treatment
- sophisticated inhalers
- drug-releasing vaginal rings and intrauterine devices (IUDs) as an effective means of long-term drug delivery in women
- dosage-adjustable self-injection devices.

Absorption processes

This chapter describes the five processes that feature in drug absorption:

- passive diffusion down a concentration gradient (most drugs)
- the cell membrane and fat-solubility of drugs (most drugs)
- active transport (few drugs)

- disintegration and dissolution of tablets (many drugs)
- presystemic metabolism (first-pass metabolism) (most drugs).

Passive diffusion down a concentration gradient

Only intravenous and inhaled anti-asthma drugs avoid the need for absorption across cell membranes. Most other drugs are absorbed from the intestine, skin and mucous membranes, mainly by passive diffusion down a concentration gradient, across cell membranes. They reach the blood capillaries by similar passive diffusion, and are distributed around the body.

The rate of absorption of a drug depends on three things: the concentration gradient, the surface area for absorption and the fat-solubility of the drug itself.

The principle of the concentration gradient is the reason why oral drugs are best absorbed if given well before a meal, as this maximises their concentration in the small intestine, from which most oral drugs are absorbed. Note the very large surface area of the jejunal villi, which makes the jejunum an ideal site for the absorption of the majority of drugs.

The cell membrane and fat-solubility of drugs

Although the cells lining many blood capillaries, particularly the kidney glomerulus, have pores between them allowing relatively free passage of drug molecules, most other tissues, including the intestine, have few intercellular pores large enough to permit drug absorption.

To be absorbed, oral drugs must therefore cross the cell membranes of the intestinal villi. As in all cells, the membrane is composed of a double layer of phospholipid, arranged like a palisade (*see* Figure 1.1). Although this is a pictorial representation, it is very close to the

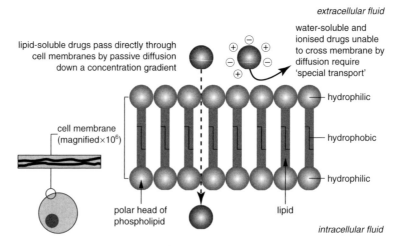

Figure 1.1 How drugs cross the cell membrane.

molecular reality revealed by the electron microscope. In essence, it means that there is a well-sealed fatty barrier between the intracellular and extracellular fluids.

Fat-soluble molecules, including some drugs, can pass directly through the cell membrane. On the right of Figure 1.1, you see that ionised and water-soluble molecules and ions, including some drugs, cannot cross the cell membrane.

Without the innate property of phospholipids to clump in this manner, cell life would be impossible, since cellular metabolism depends to a very large extent on the maintenance of strict intracellular control of water and ions such as sodium, potassium and calcium, which require active transport into and out of the cell.

An excellent example of passive diffusion and fat solubility is the almost instantaneous absorption of the anti-anginal drug glyceryl trinitrate (GTN) across the buccal mucosa. A GTN spray delivers a high concentration of this very lipid-soluble compound of very low molecular weight, which is absorbed almost as fast as an intravenous injection.

Drugs are usually formulated to make them as lipid soluble as possible, and the pharmaceutical industry has produced a variety of chemical means of achieving this end. However, sometimes a drug's low lipid solubility is used to good effect, for example, with the use of aminosalicylates in the treatment of ulcerative colitis, and the antibiotics vancomycin and neomycin. In these examples, the aim is to get the drug into the lumen of the colon for therapeutic purposes, while avoiding systemic absorption.

Many drugs are weak acids or bases (in ionic equilibrium, part ionized, part un-ionized). In such cases, only the un-ionized form is sufficiently lipid soluble to diffuse across phospholipid membranes.

Active transport across the intestinal mucosa

All cells have many active transport mechanisms. These are essential for carrying ions, most sugars, and the amino acids into and out of the cell in a highly regulated fashion, which will be described later (*see* Chapter 9).

Active transport is not a very important means of drug absorption, although iron, levodopa for Parkinson's disease, the anti-thyroid drug propylthiouracil and the anti-cancer drug fluorouracil are actively transported across the intestinal mucosa.

However, it is important to realise at this stage that active transport exists, if only because many of our most effective cardiac and other drugs act by increasing or decreasing such cellular transport mechanisms. This is what happens every time we prescribe a calcium-channel blocker, for example.

The importance of disintegration and dissolution of tablets in the stomach

Plain tablets first disintegrate and then dissolve in the stomach. Figure 1.2 shows the way in which a meal delays gastric emptying and, consequently, delays the absorption of any

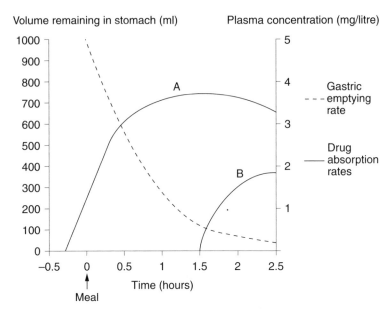

Figure 1.2 A tablet taken before a meal will dissolve in the stomach and enter the small intestine within 15 minutes (curve A); taken during or after a meal, the drug may not reach the intestine for 1–2 hours (curve B).

drug taken during or after food, and the effect that this may have on drug plasma concentration.

To achieve maximal concentration in the small intestine, where most drugs are absorbed, a drug should be taken before food. This is a simple principle about which we sometimes need reminding, particularly when prescribing most antibiotics, where achieving an adequate tissue concentration is always paramount.

In contrast, where peak plasma concentrations may be associated with side-effects, drugs can be given with food to reduce peaks.

Many modern drugs are formulated to avoid early release; for example, enteric coating is used when a drug is irritant to the gastric mucosa or when it is rendered inactive by gastric acid.

Modified-release (MR) drugs are used when the duration of action of a short-acting drug needs to be prolonged, as with the heart drug nifedipine. These formulations may also be used when a gradual rise in plasma concentration is desirable, or for patient convenience, in the hope of improving compliance.

It is essential to remember that when a branded MR product is selected for long-term therapy, as in the treatment of hypertension for example, that that branded version should always be repeated, because different MR brands of the same drug may have clinically important variations in absorption and plasma concentration. The fourteen MR nifedipine preparations are a good example of this.

Presystemic metabolism

Presystemic metabolism (breakdown of drugs by enzymes) takes place before drugs reach the systemic circulation. It occurs mainly in the liver, but a degree of breakdown also occurs in the intestinal mucosa, lungs and skeletal muscle.

Clearly, extensive metabolism results in a greatly decreased plasma concentration of drug. For example, only one-twentieth of the dose of levodopa survives first-pass metabolism in the liver, and a similar story exists for a great many drugs.

Practitioners rarely have to consider this factor, since drug dosage is designed to take into account such wastage. This explains the practical importance of bioavailability, which is the fraction of an oral dose that reaches the systemic circulation.

Why does drug absorption matter to the prescriber?

Prescribers are making decisions based on drug absorption every day. In the emergency situation, where the highest possible plasma concentration of a drug is required immediately, the drug is given intravenously, for example, intravenous furosemide (frusemide) for acute pulmonary oedema.

Intravenous injection can be difficult, for example in the treatment of an epileptic fit, when rectal administration of the highly lipid-soluble drug, diazepam, is the preferred and very effective route, as the rectum has an excellent blood supply.

Inhalers are used to deliver anti-asthmatic beta$_2$-agonists and corticosteroids directly to the lung alveoli.

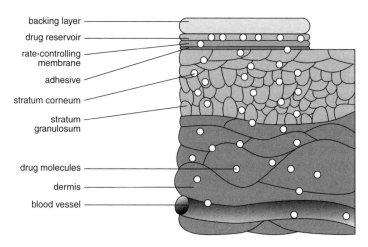

Figure 1.3 Mechanism of action of the transdermal matrix patch.

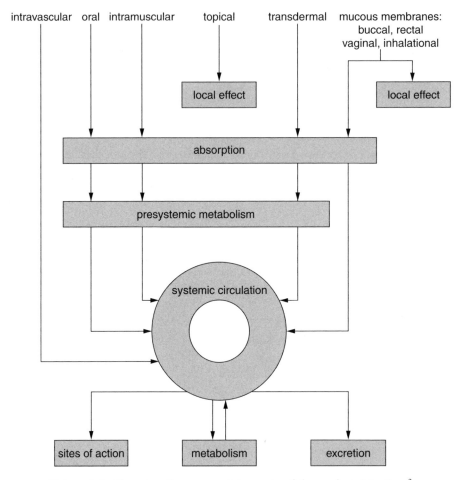

Figure 1.4 Choosing the appropriate route of drug administration.[2]

Skin conditions are usually treated by direct dermal application and of course, the transdermal route is often used for hormone replacement therapy.

Figure 1.3 shows the principle of the matrix-type skin patch. All of the drugs derived from the cholesterol stem, including the male and female sex hormones and cortisol itself, are highly lipid soluble and readily absorbed through the skin, as is fentanyl (Durogesic®), the useful strong analgesic skin patch, for managing severe chronic pain.

It is sometimes forgotten to what extent potent synthetic steroids are absorbed systemically from dermal creams, and it is important to emphasise the quantity that should be applied, for example, finger-tip units.

On the other hand, drugs that are relatively lipid insoluble, such as the antirheumatic non-steroidal anti-inflammatory drugs NSAIDs, are poorly absorbed through the skin, and are not a logical way of achieving therapeutic concentrations of anti-inflammatory agents.

Figure 1.4 summarises the routes of drug administration available to the prescriber. Which rate should be selected depends on the diagnosis, the urgency, the characteristics of the drug to be given, patient preference, and the need to avoid first-pass metabolism.

Key points

- The main principles of drug absorption are:
  - the disintegration and dissolution of tablets
  - passive diffusion down a concentration gradient
  - the cell membrane and fat-solubility of drugs
  - active transport of ions and water-soluble drugs
  - presystemic metabolism.
- Drug formulations affect absorption.
- The prescriber's aim should be the optimum drug-delivery route, i.e. the most appropriate and cost-effective.

References

1 Nachtigall LE (1995) Emerging delivery systems for estrogen replacement: aspects of transdermal and oral delivery. *Am J Obstet Gynecol.* **173**: 993-7.

2 Kruk Z and Whelpton R (1985) Focus on drug action (series). *Mims Magazine.* **January**: 44.

2 Getting a drug to its site of action: distribution

In the first chapter, we considered the principles of drug absorption from the intestine and mucous membranes, the skin and the lungs into the blood stream. The next stage in understanding drug action is to study the distribution of the absorbed drug in the blood circulating around the body, because unless a drug reaches its site of action in an adequate concentration, it will obviously not work.

Transport of drugs in the blood stream

The rate at which a drug reaches any given part of the body and the amount of drug delivered depends entirely on the rate and volume of blood perfusing that part of the anatomy (*see* Figure 2.1).

In well-perfused tissues, such as the brain, heart, kidneys and lungs (Curve 2), the concentration of drug following a bolus intravenous injection quickly reaches a maximum, which is higher than that achieved in any other tissue. Tissues in the well-perfused group will therefore achieve effective plasma concentrations relatively easily and quickly.

In tissues with intermediate rates of blood perfusion, the maximum drug concentration is lower than that in Curve 2, and is reached considerably later (Curve 3). In tissues with poor blood perfusion, such as fat, there is a prolonged delay in reaching the maximum drug concentration (Curve 4), which is lower than that in the better-perfused tissues.

Figure 2.1 represents plasma and tissue drug concentrations following intravenous injection, which is the optimal drug delivery route in terms of achieving maximal tissue concentration without first-pass metabolism. The normal route in most therapies is, of course, the oral route, in which bioavailability, i.e. the proportion of drug actually reaching the systemic circulation, is commonly reduced by incomplete intestinal absorption and first-pass metabolism in the liver.

It may be of interest to note that bioavailability is measured by comparing the area under curve (AUC) for Curve 1, resulting from the intravenous injection of a drug, with the AUC resulting from an identical oral dose.

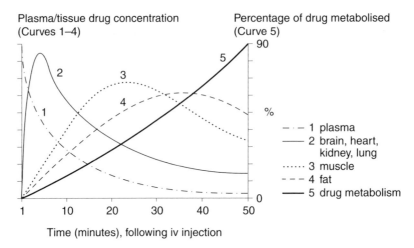

Figure 2.1 Plasma and tissue concentrations of a fat-soluble drug following bolus injection, and percentage of drug metabolised.

What happens next?

The value of Figure 2.1 is that it provides a mental picture of the entire time course of drug action. Having described the maximum concentrations in different tissues, let us follow the curves along the time axis.

Following Curve 1, why does the plasma concentration of a drug fall off so quickly? This happens for two reasons. The first is that under a positive concentration gradient, the drug passes out of the capillaries into the intercellular fluid of the body tissues until there is equilibrium between the plasma and interstitial fluid concentrations. In the intercellular fluid, the drug has access to the tissue cell receptors upon which it will exert its therapeutic effect (there is more about this topic in future chapters).

The second reason for the rapid fall in plasma concentration seen in Curve 1 (and for the progressively slower fall of tissue concentration seen in Curves 2, 3 and 4) is that on every circulation of blood through the liver, a proportion of most drugs is metabolised and usually rendered inactive. We shall consider drug metabolism and excretion in the next two chapters.

Continuing our study of Figure 2.1: how does the drug concentration in the tissues fall? Well, it is simply a reversal of the concentration gradient. As the plasma concentration (*see* Curve 1) falls due to drug metabolism (*see* Curve 5) so the concentration in the tissues comes to exceed that in the bloodstream, and the drug diffuses from the tissues back into the capillaries.

The last thing to note in Figure 2.1 is that, although the peak tissue drug concentration is lower in Curves 3 and 4, the drug remains in these tissues much longer. Likewise, the time

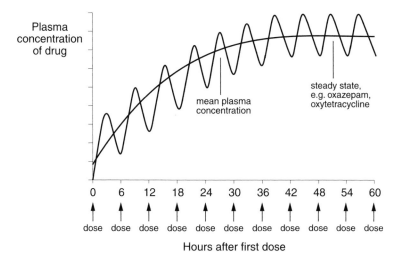

Figure 2.2 Plasma concentration of a drug with a half-life of nine hours after six-hourly oral doses – the 'steady state' concept.

taken for the tissue drug concentration to fall to half its original peak concentration (its half-life or $t_{1/2}$) is longer in Curve 3 than Curve 2, and longest of all in Curve 4.

'Steady state'

If a suitable dosage interval is chosen, the first six or seven doses will be absorbed before the preceding doses have been fully eliminated, i.e. there will be a progressive accumulation of drug in the plasma and tissues, as shown in Figure 2.2. So, for many drugs, a 'steady state' of plasma and tissue concentration is reached, typically after six or seven oral doses.

At steady state, the drug concentration in all tissues is relatively constant (input balancing output), as opposed to the scenario shown in Figure 2.1. This is why good patient compliance with dosage schedules is important.

However, drugs like amoxicillin ($t_{1/2}$ 1.5 hours) and levodopa ($t_{1/2}$ 1.5 hours) never reach steady state with normal oral dosing.

Protein binding – does it matter?

When protein bound, drugs are largely inactive. Many drugs bind loosely to plasma albumin and other proteins, but are rapidly released as free drug when their plasma concentration falls (*see* Figure 2.3).

Protein binding is only a problem when one drug, such as the heart drug verapamil, displaces another, such as digoxin, from its binding site, leading to a sudden release of free, unbound drug and possible toxicity. There are few such examples.

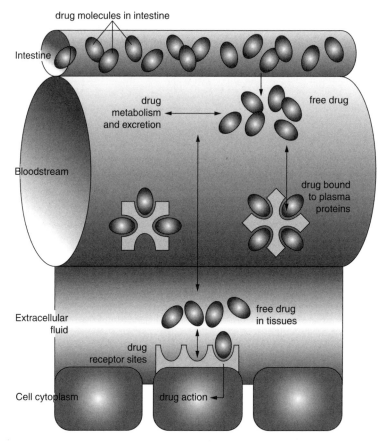

Figure 2.3 A proportion of many drugs is loosely bound to plasma proteins in the blood stream. However, this does not have a prolonged effect on the plasma concentration or drug action, as the molecules are readily released when the free drug concentration falls. Examples of drugs that are largely protein bound are: diazepam, ibuprofen, propranolol, flucloxacillin, erythromycin, phenytoin, nifedipine and verapamil.

Warfarin is 99% bound to plasma proteins, and is displaced by a number of drugs. Appendix 1 of the *British National Formulary* (*BNF*) should be consulted whenever any drug is co-prescribed with warfarin.

Hydrophilic drugs

The distribution of fat-soluble (lipophilic) drugs has been described. Water-soluble (hydrophilic) drugs show different kinetics (their absorption, distribution, metabolism and excretion):

- they are slowly and only partially absorbed

- they are not subject to significant first-pass metabolism in the liver
- they do not cross the healthy blood-brain barrier
- they are only slightly protein-bound, or not protein-bound at all
- they are filtered unchanged by the kidney, without reabsorption (*see* Chapter 4 on drug excretion). Examples of such hydrophilic drugs are the antibiotic phenoxymethylpenicillin and the heart drugs lisinopril and atenolol.

Key points

■ Distribution of a drug around the body is not uniform.

■ Well-perfused tissues receive higher drug concentrations, faster.

■ With good compliance, many drugs used for long-term maintenance therapy reach 'steady state', in which all body tissues receive a similar drug concentration.

■ Protein binding of drugs is usually not important and does not affect efficacy.

---

3 Inactivating drugs: phase 1 drug metabolism

One of the main reasons that we can use drugs as therapy, without poisoning the patient, is that the body is generally very good at inactivating and getting rid of them.

In Chapter 1, we saw that the majority of effective drugs are relatively fat soluble, since these pass easily across cell membranes during absorption from the intestinal villi and distribution around the body. In Chapter 2, we saw that more fat-soluble drugs escape more easily from the peripheral capillaries into the intercellular fluid.

Why bring up fat-solubility again? Because the most effective way of making a drug inactive or less active is often to render it more water soluble, which can be done in various ways, for example by adding an oxygen atom, (oxidation), or adding an OH^- ion (hydroxylation). This is what happens in phase 1 metabolism in the liver. How this happens is a most interesting topic that is vital to understanding the clinical problem of drug interaction, which is the cause of a significant proportion of hospital admissions due to prescribed drugs. Many of these emergencies could be avoided if all prescribers had a clear grasp of the concepts in this chapter.

CYP isoenzymes

To understand hepatic drug metabolism is to go back at least 200 million years to the original vertebrates – the fishes. In all natural environments, the food supply is contaminated to a greater or lesser extent. Ingestion of toxins from plants, rotting food, bacteria or fungi risks death from poisoning. Any animal species that can detoxify such toxins clearly has a greatly enhanced survival probability.

However, there are hundreds of environmental toxins that require many different enzymes in order to render them all inactive. Thus, over 200 million years, vertebrates have developed an extensive battery of enzymes that render toxins inactive by reducing their fat solubility (*see* Figure 3.1). This battery is the cytochrome P450 oxidase system, or CYP.

CYP is a wide range of isoenzymes of which one or more will be able to neutralise any given toxin. Figure 3.2 shows the reaction sequence of the CYP enzymes. Apart from hormones, all drugs are foreign substances (xenobiotics) and therefore potential toxins and

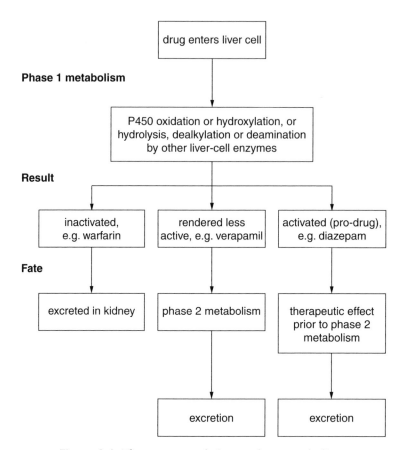

Figure 3.1 The concepts of phase 1 drug metabolism.

they are treated as such by CYP in the liver. Those drugs or poisons that the CYP system cannot metabolise are processed by other enzyme systems, also in the liver.

Figure 3.2 shows that phase 1 drug metabolism is by no means difficult to understand. Figures 3.1 and 3.2 together explain the main concepts involved.

Most of the CYP enzymes involved in drug metabolism are in the liver. They are gradually being classified into groups and subgroups, with another half dozen appearing with every year of research. It will probably be some decades before the complexity of the CYP system is fully understood. Table 3.1 gives some examples of CYP enzymes, with some of the drugs they metabolise.

P450 inhibition and induction

The inactivation of fat-soluble drugs is largely dependent on hepatic metabolism, and anything that affects this will also affect the plasma concentration of drugs. Certain drugs

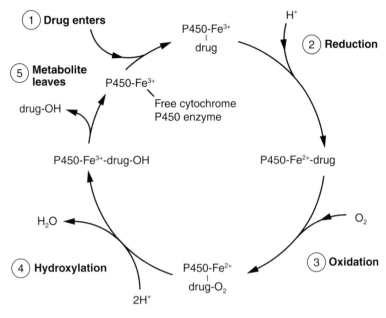

Figure 3.2 A scheme showing phase 1 hydroxylation by cytochrome P450 metabolism. The sequence of events should be read clockwise from 1–5.

disturb CYP function in one of two different, and opposite, ways: drugs may reduce CYP enzyme action (inhibition) or enhance enzyme action (induction). These effects become important when two drugs are co-prescribed, one of which inhibits or induces the CYP on which the other is dependent for its metabolism. As CYP enzymes metabolise drugs, it follows that inhibition of CYP will slow the second drug's metabolism and so lead to an increase in its plasma concentration, possibly to toxic levels. Induction of CYP, on the other hand, will speed up the second drug's metabolism and cause a reduction in its plasma concentration and potential treatment failure.

Table 3.1 Some medically important cytochrome P450 enzymes.

CYP family	Examples of drugs metabolised by this CYP family
CYP1A1	theophylline
CYP1A2	caffeine, paracetamol
CYP2C9	ibuprofen, phenytoin, warfarin
CYP2C19	omeprazole
CYP2D6	clozapine, codeine, tricyclic antidepressants
CYP3A4/5	erythromycin, losartan, nifedipine and many others

Table 3.2 Metabolic enzyme inhibitors: these *increase the effect* of drugs whose metabolism is inhibited.

Enzyme inhibitor	*Drugs affected*
imidazole antifungals, e.g. fluconazole, itraconazole, etc.	acenocoumarol (nicoumalone), alfentanil, antivirals, ciclosporin, corticosteroids, digoxin, felodipine, midazolam, phenytoin, quinidine, rifabutin, sildenafil, sulphonylureas, tacrolimus, theophylline, warfarin
cimetidine	• anthelmintics • antiarrythmics: amiodarone, flecainide, lidocaine (lignocaine), procainamide, propafenone, quinidine • antibacterials: erythromycin, metronidazole • anticoagulants: acenocoumarol, warfarin • antidepressants: amitriptyline, doxepin, moclobemide, nortriptyline • antiepileptics: carbamazepine, phenytoin, valproate • antifungals: terbinafine • antihistamines: loratadine • antimalarials: chloroquine, quinine • anxiolytics and hypnotics: benzodiazepines, clomethiazole • beta-blockers: labetalol, propranolol • calcium-channel blockers: some • cytotoxics: fluorouracil • immunosuppressant: ciclosporin (possibly) • NSAIDs: azapropazone (possibly) • opioid analgesics: pethidine • theophylline
omeprazole	diazepam, digoxin (possibly)
allopurinol	ciclosporin
erythromycin and other macrolides	alfentanil, amiodarone, bromocriptine, cabergoline, carbamazepine, ciclosporin, clozapine, disopyramide, felodipine, midazolam, rifabutin, sildenafil, terfenadine, theophylline, zopiclone
ciprofloxacin	theophylline
sulphonamides	phenytoin
amiodarone	acenocoumarol, ciclosporin, digoxin, flecainide, phenytoin, procainamide, quinidine, warfarin
metronidazole	phenytoin, fluorouracil
SSRIs	benzodiazepines (some), carbamazepine, clozapine, flecainide, haloperidol, phenytoin, propranolol, theophylline, tricyclic antidepressants
calcium-channel blockers – verapamil, diltiazem	alcohol, ciclosporin, digoxin, imipramine, midazolam, nifedipine, phenytoin, quinidine, theophylline

Note: the enzyme-inducing drugs in the left-hand column are all commonly prescribed in the community; many of those in the right-hand column are also commonly used. The potential for toxicity demands the greatest vigilance.

Table 3.3 Metabolic enzyme inducers: these *reduce the effect* of drugs whose metabolism is accelerated.

Enzyme inducer	Drugs affected
barbiturates and primidone*	acenocoumarol (nicoumalone), chloramphenicol, ciclosporin, corticosteroids, digitoxin, disopyramide, doxycycline, gestrinone, indinavir, lamotrigine, levothyroxine (thyroxine), metronidazole, mianserin, oral contraceptives, quinidine, theophylline, tibolone, toremifene, tricyclics, warfarin
phenytoin*	acenocoumarol, ciclosporin, clozapine, corticosteroids, digitoxin, disopyramide, indinavir, itraconazole, ketoconazole, lamotrigine, methadone, mexiletine, mianserin, oral contraceptives, paroxetine, quetiapine, quinidine, theophylline, thyroxine, warfarin
carbamazepine	acenocoumarol, antiepileptics, ciclosporin, corticosteroids, digitoxin, gestrinone, haloperidol, indinavir, mianserin, olanzapine, oral contraceptives, risperidone, theophylline, tibolone, toremifene, tricyclic antidepressants, warfarin
rifamycins	acenocoumarol, atovaquone, benzodiazepines, bisoprolol, carbamazepine, chloramphenicol, chlorpropamide, ciclosporin, cimetidine, corticosteroids, dapsone, digitoxin, diltiazem, disopyramide, fluconazole, fluvastatin, haloperidol, indinavir, itraconazole, ketoconazole, levothyroxine, methadone, mexiletine, nifedipine, oral contraceptives, phenytoin, propafenone, propranolol, quinidine, tacrolimus, terbinafine, theophylline, tolbutamide, tricyclic antidepressants, verapamil, warfarin
griseofulvin	acenocoumarol, ciclosporin, oral contraceptives, warfarin
alcohol	paracetamol (toxic metabolites increased), tolbutamide

* Combination therapy with two or more antiepileptic drugs enhances toxicity, and drug interactions may occur between antiepileptics (see *BNF*, Appendix 1, Antiepileptics).

Drug interaction software packages, of which there are now several versions, should be used whenever there is the slightest doubt as to the compatibility of two or more co-prescribed drugs.

Dozens of drugs are affected by these processes, and Tables 3.2 and 3.3 summarise those of greatest importance. Obviously these tables include many of our most commonly used primary care drugs. A good alternative to using drug interaction software is to have a checklist on one's desk, such as these tables, to refer to every time one of the drugs in the left-hand column is co-prescribed with another drug. A warning sticker on A4 record folders or a 'stop and check' signal on the computer record would help to prevent the harm that often occurs due to one drug's inhibition or induction of a second drug's metabolism.

Enzyme induction and inhibition are only two of the different types of drug:drug interactions that are of clinical importance. We shall consider all of them in Chapter 12.

For the sake of completeness it is worth noting that, at therapeutic doses, there is more than enough of the specific P450 enzyme available to metabolise most drugs rapidly, i.e. the metabolic processes are rarely saturated except in poisonous dosages.

Pharmacologically active phase 1 metabolites

It is also important to know that while phase 1 metabolism usually inactivates a drug or poison, in some cases the metabolite retains a pharmacological effect, although this is usually weaker than the effect of the parent drug.

In a few, but often fatal, cases the metabolite is highly toxic. Paraquat is one example of this – the metabolite releases a reactive oxygen species – and paracetamol overdose is another – the metabolite binds with liver cell macromolecules. Cell death is the result in both cases.

Quite a number of commonly-prescribed drugs are prodrugs, which are activated by phase 1 metabolism (*see* Figure 3.1). These include morphine, codeine, enalapril, amitriptyline and diazepam.

Alcohol and phenytoin

Alcohol, that ubiquitous social lubricant/drug/poison, is not metabolised by the P450 system, but by alcohol dehydrogenase and aldehyde dehydrogenase, which are also found in the liver.

The capacity of these two enzymes is limited, hence the slow metabolism of alcohol, leading to inebriation and sometimes loss of driving licence! Saturation of the enzymes occurs on consumption of 1–2 units of ethanol, after which the ethanol concentration in the plasma, and consequently the breath, rises inexorably with successive drinks.

Saturation of the enzyme that processes the antiepileptic, phenytoin, occurs at the lower therapeutic dosages, after which its plasma concentration slowly reaches toxic levels. Prescribers need to be aware of the huge individual variability in phenytoin metabolic capacity, especially in children.

Other sites of drug metabolism

All body tissues have some metabolic activity. Those with medically significant metabolic capacity include the lungs, which metabolise most prostanoids (*see* Chapter 7), the kidneys, which metabolise serotonin and norepinephrine (noradrenaline), the intestine, which metabolises salbutamol, and plasma, which metabolises suxamethonium.

In every case, extrahepatic metabolism is due to the presence of the specific metabolic enzymes in the tissue involved.

Key points

- Phase 1 drug metabolism occurs mainly via the cytochrome P450 enzyme system (CYP).
- Metabolism occurs mainly in the liver, where P450 enzymes are concentrated.
- Phase 1 metabolism makes a drug more water soluble, less able to cross cell membranes and more easily excreted.
- The chemical reactions of phase 1 are oxidation, hydroxylation, reduction and hydrolysis.
- Prodrugs are intentionally activated by phase 1 metabolism.
- Several common drugs either inhibit or induce the liver enzymes, which can lead to some of the most serious drug:drug interactions.

4 Phase 2 drug metabolism and methods of excretion

Chapters 1 and 2 described the processes and problems of getting drugs into the body and onwards to their sites of action. The processes of deactivating and eliminating drugs are also important for the prescriber, not to mention the patient!

In Chapter 3 we looked at phase 1 of drug metabolism, which involves oxidation and hydroxylation reactions, among others to inactivate the drug and render it more water soluble.

The result of the first phase of drug metabolism is that the metabolite is more easily excreted via the kidneys, which are by far the most important route of drug excretion. Many drugs are excreted unchanged in the urine, and most of the rest are excreted as phase 1 metabolites.

Drugs that require further metabolism

The phase 1 metabolites of some important drugs are not water soluble enough or polar enough for excretion, e.g. the metabolites of aspirin, morphine and methyldopa. These, and others, undergo further chemical processing in the liver, known as phase 2 metabolism.

In this phase, the drug or its phase 1 metabolite is chemically bound or conjugated to one of a number of molecules, including glucuronide, sulphate or acetyl groups, to create a larger, polarised molecule (*see* Figure 4.1).

The resulting conjugated drug is usually inactive pharmacologically, and very much more water soluble and therefore more easily excreted in urine or bile. Surprisingly, some drugs are activated by conjugation – morphine-6-glucuronide is more active than morphine itself!

A number of the body's own products are conjugated before excretion, e.g. the steroid hormones and bilirubin. Neonatal jaundice is due to the relative inability of the newborn liver to conjugate excess bilirubin.

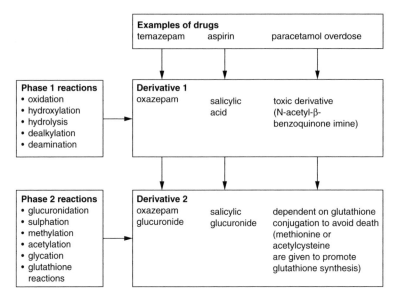

Figure 4.1 The reactions that can occur in phase 1 and 2 drug metabolism, and some examples of the products formed.

Excretion of drugs and their metabolites from the kidney

Figure 4.2 represents the function of a single renal tubule, as regards drug and metabolite excretion. Following through from left to right:

1   Approximately 20% of the drug content of blood perfusing the kidney will pass freely from the glomerulus into the renal tubule. The remaining 80% is carried in the efferent arteriole to the proximal convoluted tubule.

2   Two carrier systems in the tubular cells (one for acids, the other for bases) actively transport the drug metabolite from the capillary into the proximal tubule unidirectionally. Examples include: acetazolamide, aminosalicylate, furosemide (frusemide), indometacin, penicillins, thiazide diuretics, dopamine, morphine, quinine, serotonin, amiloride and triamterene.

3   Probenecid affects the transport of both penicillin and uric acid. It is used primarily to prolong the action of penicillin as it retards its excretion, but also in gout prophylaxis as it inhibits the reabsorption of uric acid. Sulfinpyrazone also inhibits the transport of uric acid and is used in the treatment of gout.

4   Water is then reabsorbed in the collecting duct and the drug or drug metabolite is excreted in the urine.

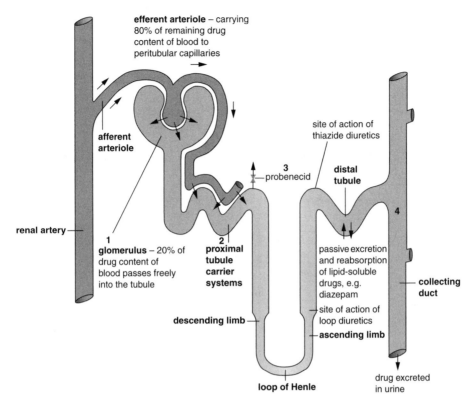

Figure 4.2 Processes involved in the renal excretion of drugs and drug metabolites; *see* text for further discussion.

The importance of renal excretion highlights the need to consider renal impairment when prescribing for elderly patients. By the age of 70, renal function is only 50% of its youthful maximum in most people. This means that the drug-excreting capacity is also reduced by around 50%. Hence the frequent warnings in the *BNF* and *MIMS* (the pharmaceutical industry's proprietary list) regarding the dosage reduction of many drugs when prescribing for elderly patients. (*See* also Chapter 10: The scientific basis of prescribing for the elderly.)

Enterohepatic cycling

Biliary excretion of drug metabolites is common, but results in only limited elimination from the body. The reason is that in the intestine, enzymes break the conjugation bond releasing free drug, a proportion of which will be reabsorbed into the circulation in its active form.

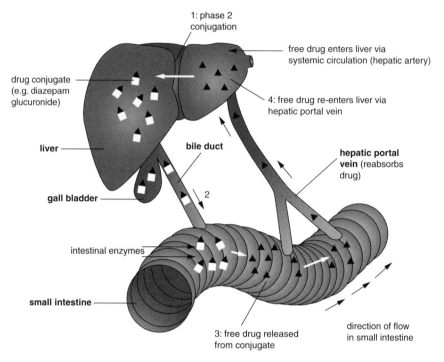

1: phase 2
conjugation

free drug enters liver via
systemic circulation (hepatic artery)

drug conjugate
(e.g. diazepam
glucuronide)

4: free drug re-enters liver via
hepatic portal vein

liver

bile duct

hepatic portal
vein (reabsorbs
drug)

gall bladder

2

intestinal enzymes

small intestine

3: free drug released
from conjugate

direction of flow
in small intestine

Figure 4.3 Enterohepatic cycling is important in the metabolism of some drugs; *see* text for further discussion.

Why mention biliary excretion at all, then? First, because it becomes an important route of excretion when renal function is poor. Second, because two commonly prescribed classes of drugs are affected – the benzodiazepines and the oral contraceptives.

Diazepam and its active metabolites are eventually conjugated as glucuronides in phase 2 reactions: *see* Figure 4.3 (1). A proportion of the diazepam glucuronide passes in the bile into the intestine (2). Intestinal enzymes split the glucuronide bond releasing free diazepam (3) which is then reabsorbed (4).

This process is called enterohepatic cycling, and is part of the reason for the very prolonged half-life of diazepam. Ultimately, most diazepam excretion occurs via the kidneys.

Enterohepatic cycling is also the reason why such low doses of oestrogen can be used in the contraceptive pill and patch. The oestrogen is repeatedly recycled (*see* Figure 4.3) and so maintains its anovulatory function.

Disruption of enterohepatic cycling explains why diarrhoea from any cause, including the therapeutic use of antibiotics, results in plasma concentrations of oestrogen inadequate to suppress ovulation. Women should be repeatedly reminded of the need to take additional precautions in such circumstances. Rapid diarrhoeal peristalsis greatly reduces the time available for enterohepatic recycling, leading to contraceptive failure, since more oestrogen is excreted.

Drugs in breast milk

Excretion of drugs in breast milk is not a maternally significant route of excretion, but may be very harmful to the breastfed baby.

Note that many of these drugs may be unavoidable – hence the importance of the prescriber's awareness of potential harm to the infant.

Table 4.1 is a useful short guide for prescribers on this topic. It would do no harm to insert a copy in the clinical record of every breastfeeding mother as a checklist in case any prescription is needed, apart from those normally given postpartum. The full source is Appendix 5 of the *BNF*.

A further problem caused by the excretion of drugs in milk is that antibiotics and other growth enhancers added to cattle feed may be excreted into cows' milk and can cause allergic responses in humans.

Table 4.1 Adverse effects of some drugs on the breastfed baby;[1] this table is not comprehensive and prescribers should consult the *BNF*, Appendix 5 when prescribing for breastfeeding women.

Maternal drug	Effect on breastfed infant
alcohol and most anxiolytics	excessive maternal ingestion may lead to drowsiness and inhibit the infant's suckling reflex
anticoagulants	risk of neonatal haemorrahge, which is increased in the presence of vitamin K deficiency, so supplements should be prescribed with the anticoagulant; warfarin appears safe
antidepressants	the MAOIs and tricyclic antidepressants are unlikely to be harmful, but are best avoided as sedation may result; fluoxetine is secreted in significant amounts and should be avoided
antiepileptics	barbiturates may lead to drowsiness, lethargy and weight loss in the infant with repeated doses; phenytoin is excreted in small amounts in breast milk, so monitoring of maternal plasma levels is important; primidone and phenobarbital may lead to drowsiness in the infant; phenobarbital and phenytoin have had reports of methaemoglobinaemia
antimanic drugs	lithium intoxication is a potential problem, although the incidence of adverse effects is low; the risk increases with continuous ingestion so maternal and, if necessary, infant plasma concentrations should be monitored and good control achieved

Table 4.1 Continued.

Maternal drug	Effect on breastfed infant
antimicrobials	
– ampicillin	the infant can develop candidosis
– benzylpenicillin	may rarely produce allergic reactions or penicillin sensitivity
– chloramphenicol	can rarely lead to aplastic anaemia and leucopenia in the infant and is best avoided
– clindamycin	bloody diarrhoea has been reported
– nalidixic acid	haemolytic anaemia has been reported
– sulphonamides and cotrimoxazole	sulphonamides can lead to kernicterus; haemolysis can occur in G6PD-deficient infants; risk of folic acid-deficiency anaemia if used long term, so haemoglobin should be checked
– tetracyclines	possibility of causing discoloration of teeth in infants
antipsychotic drugs	although excreted in small amounts in milk, antipsychotic drugs are best avoided unless absolutely necessary; animal studies indicate possible effects on the developing nervous system
antithyroid drugs	carbimazole and propylthiouracil: breastfeeding is not contraindicated provided neonatal development is closely monitored and lowest possible doses are used; breastfeeding is contraindicated if mother is taking iodine
aspirin	risk of Reye's syndrome and hypoprothrombinaemia in infants and should be avoided
atropine	atropine can have antimuscarinic side-effects in the infant
fluoride	babies of mothers drinking high-fluoride water may be at risk of developing mottled teeth
hypoglycaemic agents	use should be cautious while breastfeeding, and the infant should be monitored for hypoglycaemia
hypotensive agents	infant should be monitored; large doses of diuretics may suppress lactation
immunosuppressive drugs	breastfeeding should be discontinued
laxatives	aloe, cascara and senna are all secreted in amounts sufficient to cause purgation in the infant
oestrogen contraceptives	the oral combined pill may affect lactation itself, and so should be avoided
radiochemicals	breastfeeding is contraindicated

This concludes the prescriber's guide to pharmacokinetics – 'what the body does to drugs'. Chapters 5–9 are an introduction to pharmacodynamics – 'what drugs do to the body'.

Key points

- Some drug metabolites require further metabolism after phase 1, for example aspirin and methyldopa.
- Phase 2 metabolism conjugation reactions occur in the liver.
- Some drugs, for example morphine, are further activated by phase 2 metabolism.
- The kidneys are the most important route of drug excretion.
- Biliary excretion of drugs is less important.
- Factors affecting enterohepatic cycling, for example diarrhoea, can reduce the plasma concentration of some drugs.
- Excretion of drugs in breast milk occurs and can have an adverse effect on the breastfed infant.

Reference

1 Ledward R (1996) Safe prescribing for the breastfeeding mother. *Prescriber.* 7: 33–6.

5 Receptor function and intercellular signalling

In Chapters 1–4 we studied pharmacokinetics: the routes of administration and the processes of absorption, distribution, metabolism and excretion of drugs, with its relevance to prescribing in general practice.

We now come to a most interesting part of modern prescribing science, concerning how drugs modify the function of body organs through their effects at the level of individual cells, namely pharmacodynamics. It is here, through the advances in molecular biology, that our knowledge of drug action has expanded so greatly in the past 30 years.

Cellular society

As in human society, the infinitely complex groups of cells that form the human body succeed only so long as each individual cell participates appropriately (*see* Box 5.1).

This analogy is inadequate, however, since the cells in the healthy body live within their constraints far more precisely than humans in any human society. The individual cell exists only in the context of its society, and this has probably been the case ever since the first multicellular organisms appeared some one billion years ago.

Box 5.1 How healthy cells co-operate.

In good health each cell:

- performs its own specialised function adequately
- observes all the rules imposed upon it by the rest of the 'cellular society'
- accepts the communications (signals) from other parts of the same organ and distant organs
- interprets those signals correctly
- responds to those signals appropriately
- transmits its own signals to the other cells accurately.

Intercellular signalling

Cells communicate via chemical and electrical signalling. This is an immensely complex topic and only the chemical factors that are relevant to drug treatment will be described here. The relevant features of intercellular signalling are as follows:

- it is achieved by the secretion of a chemical molecule by the transmitting cell
- there are many chemical signalling molecules, including proteins, e.g. insulin; amino acid derivatives, e.g. noradrenaline, serotonin, thyroxine; steroids, e.g. cortisol, testosterone; fatty acid derivatives, e.g. the prostaglandins and leukotrienes; and nitric oxide
- the signalling molecule, known as the ligand, may travel far from its secreting cell, e.g. hormones (endocrine signals), may act only locally, e.g. the chemical signals controlling inflammation (paracrine signals), or may act only on a single cell across a nerve synapse, e.g. most neurotransmitters
- the 'receiving' cell recognises only the signals, or ligands, that are relevant to it: embedded in the cell membrane are a variety of proteins, some of which are receptors, with different receptors for different chemical signals
- a receptor recognises its ligand and binds it with a reversible chemical bond
- the process of chemical binding causes conformational change in the receptor protein. This change in structure activates it and leads to further signalling within the cell; the signalling in turn causes the appropriate alteration in cell function (*see* Figure 5.1 and the doorbell analogy)
- at any given moment throughout life, each of the multi-billion body cells will be receiving many different chemical signals. Each cell has been programmed to integrate these signals and to respond to all of its incoming information, producing an appropriate, graded response proportionate to the biological needs of the organ and organism.

The doorbell analogy

It is useful to consider receptors as similar to a doorbell (*see* Figure 5.1). There is a recognition site, the bell-button (2), which receives the external signal, the person ringing the bell (1). There is a transducer site, the bell-wire (3), which carries the coded signal into the cell, the house. An effector site, the bell (4), produces an entirely different signal on the inside of the cell from that which was applied on the outside. Finally, an appropriate response (5) is evoked within the cell, just as a ringing bell evokes an appropriate response within a house.

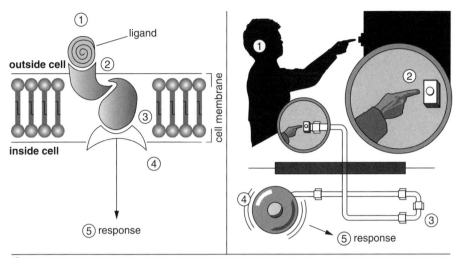

① Chemical signal (ligand) in form of drug or endogenous transmitter (person as messenger)

② Recognition site – this is the receptor protein (doorbell)

③ Transducer site – this carries the coded message into the cell (bell wire)

④ Effector site where translation of the message leads to a signal (sound of bell ringing)

⑤ Response – an appropriate action results from the signal (answering the door)

Figure 5.1 Concept of a cell receptor using the doorbell analogy.[1]

Agonists and antagonists

Many of our drugs mimic endogenous (natural) chemical signals by binding as ligands at receptors on cell membranes. Some are agonists, others are antagonists, depending on their effects at the receptor. Those drugs that initiate a response when bound to such recognition sites are called agonists, e.g. salbutamol. Natural agonists include neurotransmitters, neuromodulators, growth control factors, hormones, co-enzymes and enzymes.

Those drugs that bind to such recognition sites without causing a response, but prevent access to the site by the natural agonist, are known as antagonists or receptor blockers. These are prescribed on a daily basis, for example, the gastic acid suppressant, ranitidine.

It is important to realise that a variety of receptors are present on the surface of most cells for the purpose of receiving chemical signals.

Receptor-linked ion channels

In the receptor-linked ion channel, the recognition site, transducer site and effector are combined in one complex protein molecule. Figure 5.2 shows how skeletal muscle

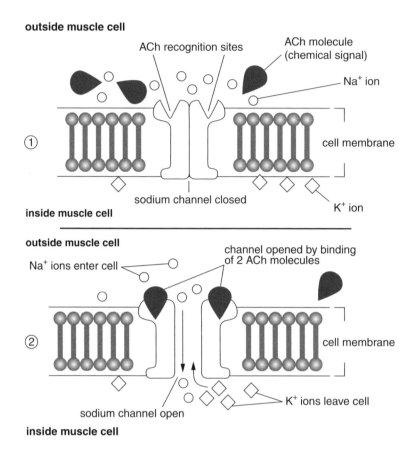

Figure 5.2 Example of a receptor-linked ion channel in skeletal muscle; the closed ion channel (1) opens in response to ACh binding (2), which leads to depolarisation of the muscle cell and initiation of contraction.[1]

contraction is triggered via sodium ion channels. The sodium channel is a protein that is directly linked to the acetylcholine (ACh) receptor and remains closed to ions except on stimulation under strict regulation. This stimulation comes in the form of a chemical signal, in this case ACh molecules released from a motor neurone into the synaptic cleft.

Binding of the ACh molecule to the recognition site causes conformational change in the protein that forms the walls of the sodium channel (the transducer) and opens the sodium channel (the effector). Sodium ions enter the muscle cell, causing depolarisation and consequent muscle contraction (the response).

Several important muscle relaxants used in anaesthesia, e.g. pancuronium and atracurium, block the binding of ACh to the recognition site of sodium channels in skeletal muscle.

Receptors linked to enzymes

The other type of effector associated with receptors is the enzyme. In Figure 5.3, note the chemical signal binding to the recognition site. This causes the transducer to activate the effector via a regulatory subunit. The effector is adenylate cyclase, which converts adenosine triphosphate (ATP) in the cell to cyclic adenosine monophosphate (cyclic AMP).

Cyclic AMP is an important intracellular secondary messenger, which rapidly diffuses from the membrane into the cytoplasm where it triggers a series of metabolic events leading to the final response within the cell.

Many drugs exert their effects via enzyme-linked receptors (*see* Table 5.1) and some via ion channels (*see* Table 5.2).

Many receptors involve activation of a protein known as the G-protein, which is an intermediate chemical messenger. This then controls the activation or inhibition of a specific effector. There are two other 'families' of receptors, which will not be described at present.

Amplifying the signal

One important feature of receptors with enzyme system effectors is the capacity for amplification of the original chemical signal. One extracellular signal at the recognition

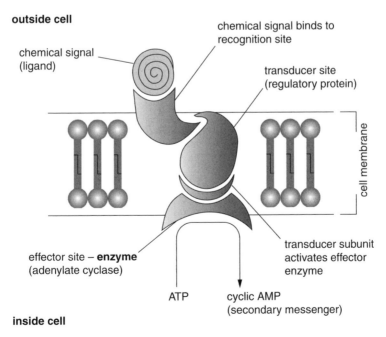

Figure 5.3 Concept of an enzyme-linked receptor (highly diagrammatic).[1]

Table 5.1 Receptor agonists using adenylate cyclase as the effector in disease processes, and the drugs that treat them (S indicates stimulation of cyclic AMP production and I indicates inhibition).

	Agonist	*Disease involving this agonist*	*Drug treatment*
S	dopamine	schizophrenia – excessive dopamine	phenothiazine antipsychotics, e.g. chlorpromazine, haloperidol, fluphenazine
		Parkinson's disease – loss of dopamine neurones	levodopa and dopamine agonists, e.g. pergolide
		hyperprolactinaemia – dopamine deficit	bromocriptine
		chemically and radiologically induced nausea, GI disorders involving spasticity, migraine, nausea	metoclopramide
S	noradrenaline	hypertension, angina	beta-blockers, methyldopa
S	adrenaline	asthma	salbutamol, terbutaline and occasionally adrenaline itself
S	serotonin	migraine	sumatriptan
		depression	SSRIs
S	histamine	H_1 – inflammation (allergic), motion sickness	antihistamines, cyclizine
		H_2 – peptic ulceration	H_2-receptor antagonists
I	prostaglandins	inflammatory disease, particularly in joints	NSAIDs
S	glucagon	hypoglycaemia	glucagon
S	vasopressin	diabetes insipidus	vasopressin analogues
I	angiotensin-II	hypertension	angiotensin-II receptor antagonists
I	endogenous opiates	severe pain	opioid analgesics

Table 5.2 Drugs that exert their effect via receptor-linked ion channels.

Ion channel	Site	Drug	Effect
GABA-linked receptors	throughout brain	all barbiturates, all benzodiazepines	from sedation to anaesthesia
5-HT$_3$ receptors (serotonin)	vomiting centre in medulla, GI tract	ondansetron, granisetron, tropisetron, etc.	powerful antiemetics used in chemotherapy
nicotinic ACh receptors	all skeletal muscle (at the neuromuscular junction)	pancuronium, vercuronium, etc.	powerful muscle relaxants used in anaesthesia

site can generate thousands of end-products; an example of this is the glycogen cascade in the liver leading to the formation of glucose. Such explosive responses require tight regulation, and in all cells there are efficient mechanisms for rapidly degrading the enzyme effectors such as cyclic AMP.

It is also useful to appreciate the speed of these biochemical reactions – fractions of a second in many cases.

A similar cascade causes synthesis of the prostaglandins, which are very important medically; this will be described in detail in Chapter 7. The prostaglandins are important physiological regulators but are also involved in destructive inflammatory processes.

How is the chemical signal switched off?

The majority of signal molecules are broken down (metabolised), usually by specific local enzymes, soon after binding with their receptor. This usually leads to a cessation of the intracellular response.

In the case of neurotransmitters such as noradrenaline, acetylcholine, serotonin and dopamine, the breakdown occurs in milliseconds. Excess neurotransmitter is often re-absorbed by the transmitting neurone (as, for example, with serotonin reuptake). Local paracrine signals are broken down enzymatically within minutes, as, for example, with the prostaglandins. However, some true hormones such as cortisol and thyroxine are not broken down for many hours.

Conclusion

This article has briefly covered the fundamental concepts of receptor theory. This includes where receptors are located, how the two main types of receptors work, how endogenous and exogenous chemical messengers (drugs) may activate or block receptors, and how this chemical message at the cell surface is changed to a quite different signal within the cell, sometimes with great amplification, altering cell function.

Key points

- The human body functions only because of tight regulation of all its individual cells.
- Regulation is achieved by continuous intercellular signalling.
- All cells both transmit and receive signals.
- The actual signals are chemical molecules such as noradrenaline, insulin, serotonin and prostaglandins.
- The cell receives the chemical signal at a receptor.
- The receptor is often a specialised protein in the cell membrane.
- The receptor recognition site is linked to an effector that initiates metabolic or ionic change within the cell.
- The effector is often an enzyme or ion channel.
- Many commonly-used drugs block or stimulate these receptors.

Reference

1 Kruk Z and Whelpton R (1985) Focus on drug action. *Mims Magazine.* **April:** 67.

Further reading

- Alberts B *et al.* (eds) (1994) *Molecular Biology of the Cell.* (3e). Garland Publishing, New York and London.
- Baynes J and Dominiczak M (1999) *Medical Biochemistry.* Mosby, London.

6 The central role of receptors in drug action

Continuing our exploration of receptor function and its relevance to the prescriber, it is well known that for any given intercellular signal, e.g. noradrenaline, there are a variety of different receptors, each type having a different, and sometimes opposite, function to the others. Figure 6.1 is a representation of different noradrenergic receptors and their functions in various tissue and neuronal sites.

The main purpose of this chapter is to remind readers that the response evoked by any given agonist or antagonist depends entirely on the type of receptor to which it binds.

Noradrenaline as a physiological agonist

Figure 6.1 shows the release of noradrenaline (NA) from a neurone across a synapse. Noradrenaline may act on $beta_1$, $beta_2$, $alpha_1$ or $alpha_2$ receptors on the postsynaptic membrane of another neurone, smooth muscle cell or cardiac muscle fibre. Each of these receptors will cause a different response in the cell when noradrenaline binds to it.

For example, in vascular smooth muscle, noradrenaline acts on $alpha_1$ receptors and causes vasoconstriction. In the smooth muscle of the bronchioles, noradrenaline acts on $beta_2$ receptors to cause relaxation.

In cardiac muscle, $beta_1$ receptors predominate and noradrenaline or adrenaline binding here will cause an increase in the rate and force of cardiac contraction.

Note the $alpha_2$ adrenergic autoreceptor in Figure 6.1. It may seem strange that a nerve ending should have built-in receptors for its own transmitter chemical. These serve as a negative feedback loop, i.e. the autoreceptors are inhibitory, and if there is a build-up of noradrenaline in the synaptic cleft, $alpha_2$ autoreceptors will inhibit further release from the neurone.

In the central nervous system (CNS), neurotransmitter action is rapidly terminated by metabolism via a specific enzyme. An example of this is monoamine oxidase (MAO), which diffuses from the surface of neuronal mitochondria and renders noradrenaline inactive. All chemical signals are metabolised to terminate their actions.

Using adrenoceptors as an example, Table 6.1 summarises their main physiological and

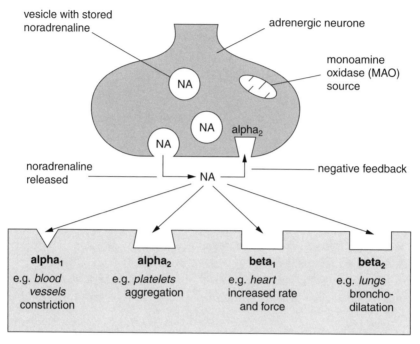

Figure 6.1 Several different receptors may exist for the same agonist; the response elicited to the agonist in a tissue or neurone depends on which receptors are present.

therapeutic effects and emphasises the importance of the receptor type and its location. The predominant receptor type in any tissue will determine the effect of the chemical signal, whether it is endogenous or a drug.

Receptor diversity

Although this chapter has concentrated on adrenoceptors by way of explaining the importance of the receptor rather than the chemical signal, receptors for most other physiological intercellular signals show similar, or even greater, diversity of response. The biological rationale is that a limited repertoire of chemical signals can be made to perform a very wide variety of functions.

Do not expect the nomenclature to be uniform either, as it is often based on the historical background of the original scientific discovery and is very confusing, as Box 6.1 demonstrates.

The purpose of Box 6.1 is first to reinforce the concept that all of these subtypes may have different physiological functions, and second, to stress again that the action of any given drug depends largely on which receptor site it occupies.

Table 6.1 The effects of noradrenaline binding to different receptor types; the italics show examples of diseases whose drug treatment involves these receptors.

Tissue	Alpha$_1$	Alpha$_2$	Beta$_1$	Beta$_2$
Smooth muscle				
blood vessels	constrict (*hypertension*)	constrict (*hypertension*)	dilate	
bronchi	constrict (*asthma*)			dilate
GI tract non-sphincter	relax (hyperpolaris-ation)			relax (no hyperpolaris-ation)
sphincter	contract			
uterus	contract			relax
bladder				
detrusor				relax
sphincter	contract (*urinary obstruction*)			
seminal tract	contract			relax
iris (radial)	contract			
ciliary muscle				relax
Heart			increased rate increased force (*angina, hypertension, heart failure*)	
Skeletal muscle				tremor
Liver	glycogenolysis K$^+$ release			glycogenolysis
Fat			lipolysis (β_3 receptor)	
Nerve terminals				
adrenergic		decreased neuro-transmission	increased neurotrans-mission	
cholinergic (some)		decreased neuro-transmission		
Salivary gland	K$^+$ release		amylase secretion	
Platelets		aggregation		
Mast cells				inhibited histamine release

Box 6.1 Different receptors for common physiological signals (ligands), which are often the targets for intervention during medical drug treatment.

Cholinergic receptors (binding acetylcholine) are subdivided into muscarinic (M) receptors and nicotinic receptors. The muscarinic receptors are divided into M_1 (neural), M_2 (cardiac) and M_3 (glandular).

Histamine receptors are subdivided into H_1 (bronchiolar, uterine and intestinal smooth muscle), H_2 (the gastric acid-secreting cells) and H_3 (neural tissue).

Serotonin receptors are of four types: $5\text{-}HT_1$ to $5\text{-}HT_4$, with several subdivisions of types $5\text{-}HT_1$ and $5\text{-}HT_2$.

Dopamine receptors are even more confusingly classified: there are two main types – D_1 and D_2, but D_1 is subdivided into D_1 and D_5, while D_2 is subdivided into D_2, D_3 and D_4.

This multiplicity of receptors is the reason why some of our most important drugs have multiple, often unwanted, side-effects, as with, for example, the beta-blockers (bronchospasm, cold feet), the tricyclic antidepressants (dry mouth, blurred vision, constipation, micturition problems, etc.) and the SSRIs (nausea, vomiting, dyspepsia, diarrhoea, constipation).

We have spent some time considering receptors and their functions because they are fundamental to the understanding of a large part of therapeutic drug use.

Some of the early drugs were the body's own natural agonists, such as adrenaline, which was used to relax the bronchioles in asthma.

However, as we have seen, the body utilises a few common chemicals but provides them with multiple actions by having different subtypes of receptor in various concentrations in different tissues. Thus, if we try to use these physiological agonists as drugs we cannot control their activity. Hence adrenaline given to relax the bronchioles in an asthma attack will also stimulate the heart, which can be dangerous.

However, as our understanding and discovery of the variety of receptors grew we developed drugs that were selective or relatively selective for different subtypes of receptor. Our understanding of receptor subtypes has revolutionised pharmacotherapy over the past 50 years.

Agonists

Although receptors are designed to be activated by endogenous ligands, they can also be activated by other molecules, particularly those with a similar structure. Armed with this knowledge, and the fact that receptors are divided into subtypes, pharmacologists set out to develop drugs that could selectively activate receptor subtypes.

A classic example of this process was the development of isoprenaline, a drug that acted as an agonist at beta adrenergic receptors but not at alpha receptors. Following the discovery that beta-receptors were divided into $beta_1$ and $beta_2$ subtypes, and that $beta_2$ receptors relaxed the bronchioles, the $beta_2$ selective agonist salbutamol was developed. Salbutamol has been a mainstay of asthma treatment ever since. Another example of agonist drugs that act on receptors are dopamine agonists, which are used in the treatment of Parkinson's disease.

Antagonists/blockers

As well as being activated by non-endogenous drugs, receptors can also be blocked. Molecules that attach to receptors but fail to elicit a response are called antagonists. They exert their effects by blocking the action of endogenous ligands. More drugs are antagonists or blockers than agonists.

A parallel example of the therapeutic development of antagonist drugs is the initial use of the beta-blocker propranolol to slow the heart in angina. As this drug blocks both $beta_1$ and $beta_2$ receptors it can also provoke bronchoconstriction. As a result, drugs like atenolol were developed that are selective blockers of the $beta_1$ receptor, and spare the bronchial $beta_2$ receptors.

Selectivity is relative

Prescribers need to be clear that receptor selectivity of drugs is relative, not absolute. 'Selective' $beta_1$ antagonists have limited action on $beta_2$ receptors, so can precipitate severe asthma. The same applies to the selective cyclo-oxygenate enzyme 2 (COX-2) inhibitor NSAIDs, which still carry some risk of GI side-effects (*see* Chapter 7).

Up- and down-regulation

Receptors are not fixed in either number or the response they elicit and thus can change during long-term stimulation or blockade. In the case of agonists like salbutamol, the response to a given drug concentration is diminished, possibly by some form of receptor desensitisation. This is called down-regulation, which has several possible mechanisms.

The reverse occurs on continual receptor blockade. The continued blockade of a receptor by drugs like beta-blockers causes receptor hypersensitivity to the physiological agonist, in this case adrenaline and noradrenaline. This up-regulation appears to be due to the synthesis of extra receptors or a shortening of the refractory phase that some receptors exhibit.

Key points

■ For a given ligand there are a variety of receptors, each of which has a different function, initiating a different cellular response.

■ Drug agonists stimulate receptor action, and antagonists inhibit it.

■ The variety of receptors can lead to unwanted adverse effects following non-specific drug agonist or antagonist treatment.

■ The newer selective agonists and antagonists are not absolute in their selectivity, and can still cause unwanted effects.

■ Long-term drug treatment can lead to up- or down-regulation of receptors, and therefore enhanced or reduced responsiveness.

7 Drugs that block enzymes: understanding NSAID therapy in inflammation

In Chapter 5 on intercellular signalling and receptors, we saw how a stimulatory chemical signal often releases a rapid cascade of enzymes in the receptive cell. This release of enzymes triggers a variety of biochemical changes within the cell. One of the best understood cascades is that leading to the production of eicosanoids: prostaglandins, leukotrienes, prostacyclins and thromboxanes.

The importance of the eicosanoids can hardly be over-emphasised. Not only are they vital in the physiological regulation of many body functions, including those of the stomach, lungs, kidneys, brain, heart and genitourinary system, but they are also key players in inflammation of all types. It is in that latter role that their immense clinical importance lies.

Non-steroidal anti-inflammatory drugs (NSAIDs), which affect the cascade, are frequently used in general practice to control inflammation. Therefore it is important to understand how they act and why they often give problems: 30% of all serious adverse drug reactions reported annually to the UK Committee on Safety of Medicines (CSM) are due to NSAIDs alone.

Revising inflammation

Inflammation is normally a protective process, triggered by mechanical or microbial damage to a variety of cells – mast cells, white cells, phagocytes, lymphocytes, platelets, etc. These cells respond to damage by producing chemical signals that mediate inflammation. The chemical signals produced include some prostaglandins, histamine, various kinins, the complement system, cytokines and platelet activating factor. Box 7.1 summarises the process involved in inflammation.

All of the changes in Box 7.1 are triggered by sophisticated and controlled chemical signalling between cells, using several or all of the chemical signals mentioned above.

Let us now focus on the prostanoids. All of the components involved in the cascade are synthesised in many body cells from phospholipid in the cell membrane itself (*see* Figure 7.1) and the raw material in this process is arachidonate. Figure 7.1 is worth a

---

Box 7.1 The process of inflammation.

Mediators of inflammation cause:

- vasodilatation, i.e. local reddening and heat; hypotension and shock can occur if widespread
- increased capillary permeability, which causes protein loss from capillaries and tissue swelling
- monocyte accumulation, which prolongs inflammation and inactivates foreign matter
- stimulation of sensory receptors, i.e. itch and pain, with protective functions
- fever, by stimulation of the hypothalamic temperature-regulation centre
- contraction of smooth muscle in the bronchioles, causing allergic asthma and, in the intestine, leading to GI pain in food allergies.

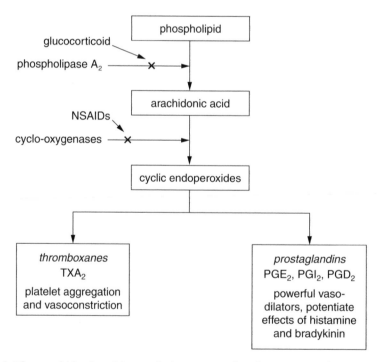

Figure 7.1 The arachidonic acid cascade is an example of an enzyme-driven pathway; the diagram shows several points where drugs block the cascade, so reducing the production of inflammatory signals.

moment's study, since it shows where current drugs interfere at different points in the enzymatic cascade.

Stimuli, such as an antigen/antibody reaction, cause an enzyme in the cytosol, phospholipase A_2, to activate. In its active form it catalyses the release of arachidonic acid from the cell membrane phospholipid into the cell.

Figure 7.1 shows why corticosteroids are such powerful anti-inflammatory agents: they block the process at step 1. In effect, they 'switch off the power at the mains'.

Once arachidonic acid has been produced, it can be used as the raw material, or substrate, for a variety of inflammatory mediators.

The prostanoids – prostaglandins and thromboxanes

As shown in Figure 7.1, arachidonic acid is metabolised by cyclo-oxygenase enzymes (COX-1 and COX-2) to an intermediate step (endoperoxide), which can be converted by one of two further enzymatic pathways to prostaglandins or thromboxanes. The inflammatory response is always accompanied by prostaglandin release; several prostaglandins cause potent vasodilatation of arterioles, pre-capillary sphincters and venules in many tissues.

The prostaglandins are by no means only pathological – they are part of the physiological regulation of blood flow. They also inhibit gastric acid secretion and have other physiological functions in many tissues.[1] However, in disease they can cause trouble, nowhere more so than in the joints.

COX-1 is found in most tissues and is involved in a variety of physiological roles. COX-2, however, is only found in inflammatory cells on activation. Therefore, COX-2 specific NSAIDs are associated with fewer unwanted effects. However, there does appear to be a trade-off as there is increasing evidence of serious side-effects with COX-2 NSAIDs, so the decision to use these drugs should not be taken lightly.

The positive and negative effects of prescribing NSAIDs

The NSAIDs, including aspirin, all inhibit the COX-1 and COX-2 enzymes. The positive result is a dramatic reduction of joint inflammation, pain and platelet aggregation. The reduction of thromboxane A_2 (TXA_2) caused by most NSAIDs is the reason for the powerful anti-thrombotic effect of even 75 mg aspirin daily.

On the negative side, most of the side-effects of the NSAIDs are due to their disruption of the prostaglandins' widespread physiological functions. In the stomach, PGE_2 inhibits acid secretion and has a protective effect on the mucosa. Therefore, the effect of NSAIDs (via COX-1) in the stomach is increased likelihood of erosion by gastric acid – the cause of NSAID-induced gastritis and peptic ulceration.

When renal circulation is impaired, prostaglandins are important in maintaining renal tubular blood flow and tubular function. That is why giving NSAIDs to elderly people with poor renal function sometimes leads to sudden deterioration of renal function and should be avoided or minimised. Box 7.2 shows the list of serious unwanted side-effects resulting from NSAID use at normal dosages.

Completing the eicosanoid picture

A moment's study will show that Figure 7.1 is included in Figure 7.2, as the left-hand pathway 1. Figure 7.2 reveals how much more complex the chemical signalling of inflammation is, by including the leukotrienes, the chemotaxins and platelet activating factor (PAF). It is clear that we have a long way to go before we have the full range of drugs needed to control this complex jigsaw.

The leukotrienes and asthma

Continuing with Figure 7.2, if arachidonate is processed by lipoxygenase (pathway 2), the end product may be a leukotriene. Like the prostaglandins, there are several leukotrienes, mostly with a physiological function. But leukotrienes are also potent mediators of inflammation – they cause 1000-fold more exudation of plasma from post-capillary venules than equivalent concentrations of histamine! The cysteinyl leukotrienes also cause intense bronchoconstriction, again far more potent in their effects than histamine. The leukotrienes may also be the 'slow-reacting substance' of anaphylaxis.

The innovation of the pharmaceutical industry has provided us with two leukotriene receptor antagonists – montelukast and zafirlukast, blocking the effects of leukotrienes in the airways. These are already useful as add-on therapy for patients with mild-to-moderate

---

Box 7.2 The main serious adverse drug reactions of NSAIDs.

- Gastritis and peptic ulceration.
- Precipitation of acute renal failure.
- Loss of antihypertensive control.
- Deterioration of chronic heart failure.
- Exacerbation of inflammatory bowel disease.
- Exacerbation of quiescent gout (in patients taking probenecid).
- Skin reactions (particularly reactivation of psoriasis).
- Loss of anticoagulation control.

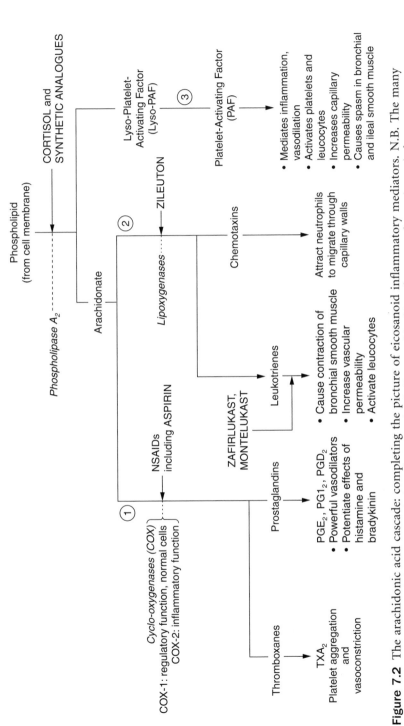

Figure 7.2 The arachidonic acid cascade: completing the picture of eicosanoid inflammatory mediators. N.B. The many physiological functions of the eicosanoids have been omitted. Enzyme-blocking drugs are shown in capitals.

asthma which is not controlled with an inhaled corticosteroid and a short-acting beta$_2$ stimulant. We are still in the early stages of leukotriene antagonist use in medicine, and it may be that the Churg-Strauss syndrome, the worrying adverse drug reaction comprising eosinophilia, vasculitic rash, worsening pulmonary systems, cardiac complications and peripheral neuropathy, may be due to the fact that our existing drugs are upsetting the balance of as yet unknown leukotriene regulation of normal function elsewhere in the body.

A new enzyme-blocking drug, zileuton, has been available for several years in the USA. This blocks the lipoxygenases, so preventing the synthesis of the leukotrienes and chemo-taxins (pathway 2 of Figure 7.2).

The pharmaceutical industry is currently researching pathway 3 of Figure 7.2 for a drug which might attenuate the powerful inflammatory effects of PAF (a major mediator of acute and chronic inflammation), including allergies.

How the corticosteroids control inflammation

When inflammation is uncontrollable by NSAIDs, as often happens in severe asthma, inflammatory bowel disease and rheumatoid arthritis, high potency synthetic steroids like

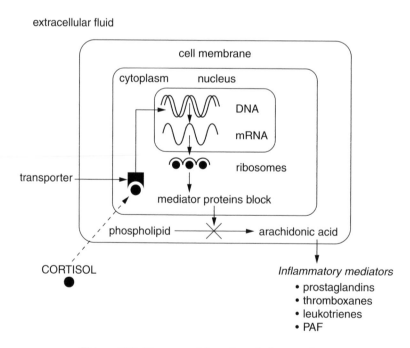

Figure 7.3 How steroids reduce inflammation.

prednisolone, betamethasone and dexamethasone are given orally. Cortisol and its many synthetic analogues act in a quite different way from all the drugs we have so far considered (*see* Figure 7.3). Steroids enter the tissue cell and are carried by a transporter molecule into the nucleus, where they activate segments of DNA to produce mRNA. This results in the production of mediator proteins at cellular ribosomes, and these proteins block the arachidonic acid cascade at its earliest point blocking the production of all the eicosanoid inflammatory mediators (*see* Figure 7.2).

Unfortunately, prolonged steroid use leads to widespread steroid side-effects, including hypertension, fluid retention and depression of the immune system. That is why more specific and powerful anti-inflammatory drugs are so eagerly awaited.

Other enzyme-blocking drugs

The NSAID story is the classic introduction to the drug manipulation of enzymatic cascades. The pharmaceutical industry has successfully targeted several quite different enzymatic processes, which community and hospital prescribers are now frequently manipulating to great benefit in some common and serious diseases.

The most obvious examples are the angiotensin converting enzyme (ACE) inhibitors in the treatment of heart failure and hypertension: these block the enzymatic conversion of the inactive substrate, angiotensin I, to the potent vasoconstrictor, angiotensin II (*see* Chapter 8).

Recently we have seen the introduction of the 5 alpha-reductase inhibitor, finasteride, a major advance in the management of benign prostatic hyperplasia (BPH): it blocks the conversion of testosterone to the more potent dihydrotestosterone.

A major advance has been the advent of the aromatase inhibitors, anastrozole, letrozole and exemestane, for advanced oestrogen-dependent breast cancer: they inhibit the enzyme responsible for the synthesis of oestrogen in post-menopausal women.

Lastly, there is the relatively selective monoamine oxidase-A inhibitor, moclobemide, for major depression, which reversibly inhibits the metabolism of 5-HT, noradrenaline and dopamine in cells of the CNS.

Chapter 8 will summarise the current targets for drug action.

Key points

- Regulatory chemical signals between cells must be synthesised within the transmitter cell.
- This synthesis usually involves one or more enzyme-dependent steps.
- There is often an enzymatic cascade in which the same starting point (substrate) may undergo one of several enzymatic conversions, resulting in different intercellular signals.
- The production of the prostaglandins, leukotrienes, thromboxanes and prostacyclins is a good example of this.
- Drugs that block such enzymes halt production of the products of that part of the cascade.
- In the case of the NSAIDs, this provides powerful anti-inflammatory medications.
- Understanding such enzymatic intracellular pathways led to the discovery of drugs that block the chemical signal themselves, for example the leukotriene receptor blockers in add-on asthma prophylaxis.
- A further development is that of the prostaglandin analogues for therapeutic use, particularly in obstetrics, gastric acid-related disease and neonatology.
- Modern treatment of advanced breast cancer, BPH, severe depression, heart failure and hypertension involve drugs that block other enzyme processes.

Reference

1 Rang HP, Dale MM and Ritter JM (1999) *Pharmacology*. Churchill Livingstone, London.

8 The principal targets for drug action

Not all drugs act by stimulating or blocking receptors or, as in the case of NSAIDs, enzymes. In fact, there are four main targets for drug action:

- receptors
- ion channels
- enzymes
- carrier molecules.

Figures 8.1–8.4 illustrate the differences between these drug targets, and relate to Chapters 5–7.

In each of these four cases, most drugs are effective because they bind to particular target proteins. This specificity is reciprocal: individual classes of drug bind only to certain targets, and individual targets recognise only certain classes of drug.

However, no drugs are completely specific in their actions, which is the reason for the unwanted side-effects of commonly used drugs.

For example, selective beta$_1$ blockers retain some beta$_2$ blockade activity and therefore remain a risk to asthmatic patients. Likewise, selective COX-2 NSAIDs retain some COX-1 activity and hence carry the risk of all of the NSAID adverse effects, although this risk is smaller than with the non-selective NSAIDs. COX-2 NSAIDs may also lack some of the beneficial side-effects of the non-selective NSAIDs.

Receptors as targets for drug therapy (see Figure 8.1)

Basic receptor theory has already been covered in Chapter 5. Since prescribers are frequently targeting receptors, it is worth looking a little further at what is currently known.

Receptors can be divided into four main subtypes, each of which relates quite closely to its physiological function:

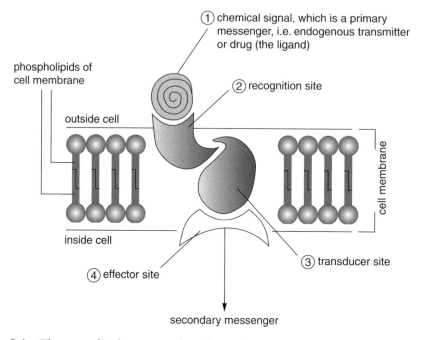

Figure 8.1a The generalised concept of a cell-membrane receptor demonstrates the process behind three of the four receptor subtypes: the drug binds to the receptor complex, triggering a series of chain reactions before the response is effected.

tissue cell

Figure 8.1b Steroid drugs are able to exploit nuclear receptors, the fourth receptor subtype, which acts directly on DNA and affects protein synthesis.

1 The ion-channel-linked cell membrane receptor. These tend to serve fast neurotransmitters in the CNS. They function in milliseconds, and are exemplified by the GABA-linked chloride ion channels where the benzodiazepines act.

2 The enzyme-linked cell membrane receptor, which is directly coupled to its enzyme. These channels produce their effects within minutes, and are exemplified by the insulin receptors.

3 The enzyme-linked cell membrane receptor, which is indirectly coupled via a G-protein. These produce their effects within seconds and serve many hormones and slow neurotransmitters, e.g. the adrenoceptors in the CNS.

4 Nuclear receptors linked to gene transcription, which are coupled via DNA. These produce their effect very slowly, over a period of hours or even days. Steroid hormones, oestrogens and thyroxine are examples of drugs that affect nuclear receptors, *see* Figure 8.1b.

Endogenous hormones and some drugs pass through the cell membrane and attach to receptors in the cytoplasm. The receptor plus ligand complex then moves across the nuclear membrane into the nucleus. Once inside the nucleus it binds to specific parts of chromosomal DNA, resulting in messenger RNA production and protein synthesis (*see*

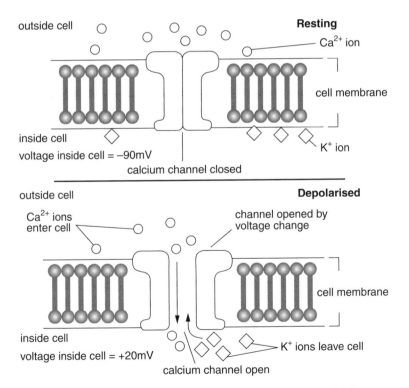

Figure 8.2 Voltage-gated ion channels open in response to a change in the voltage of the cell membrane; cardiac calcium-channel blockers, such as verapamil, block this channel.

Figure 8.1b). Steroids, oestrogen and thyroxine act via nuclear receptors, and tamoxifen blocks intracelluar oestrogen receptors.

Ion channels as targets for drug action (see Figure 8.2)

Many ion channels react to electrical rather than chemical signals. Such voltage-gated ion channels open and close in response to changes in the voltage across the cell membrane. Calcium channels in cardiac muscle are important examples (*see* Chapter 9).

Enzymes as targets for drug action

Many of our most important and powerful modern drugs act on enzymes in the plasma or inside cells. Their action is usually via enzyme blockade and examples include the

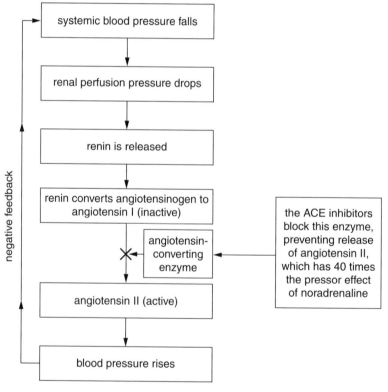

Figure 8.3 ACE inhibitors, an example of drugs that target enzymes, inhibit the production of angiotensin II, and so prevent blood pressure rising further in hypertension.

angiotensin-I converting enzyme (ACE) inhibitors (*see* Figure 8.3). All prescribers need to be aware of the function of these important drugs.

Another commonly prescribed group of enzyme blockers are the NSAIDs, whose action and adverse drug reactions were considered in the previous chapter.

The statins are another example of enzyme-inhibiting drugs. These drugs are very valuable in cardiovascular prophylaxis and their action is now well understood. The statins competitively inhibit an important enzyme involved in cholesterol synthesis in the liver (HMG-CoA). This action effectively lowers LDL-cholesterol with fewer side-effects than the older lipid-lowering agents. The statins have been proved to reduce the risk of heart attack and death in patients with angina.

Allopurinol is useful in the treatment of chronic gout because it blocks the enzyme xanthine oxidase, which catalyses the final breakdown of purines to form uric acid.

A further example of enzyme-blocking drugs is the monoamine-oxidase inhibitor (MAOI) group, which are still used occasionally in cases of depression that have not responded to other agents. The serious side-effects of the MAOIs are well known, and are due to blockade of the enzyme outside the CNS.

Carrier molecules as targets for drug action

As mentioned earlier in the book, ions and less lipid-soluble molecules are transported in and out of cells by carrier proteins. These carrier molecules play an important role in the

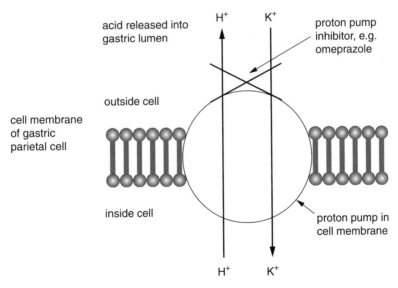

Figure 8.4 Omeprazole, which is a proton-pump inhibitor, inhibits carrier molecules transporting ions in and out of cells in the gastric mucosa, and hence prevents acid release.

Table 8.1 Some commonly used drugs and their targets.

Target	Exemplary drug and its effect on the target	
Receptor	**Agonist**	**Antagonist**
beta receptor	dobutamine	beta-blockers, e.g. propranolol
histamine H_2 receptor	histamine	ranitidine, etc.
opiate receptor	morphine	naloxone
5-HT_3 receptor	serotonin	ondansetron, etc.
dopamine D_2 receptor	dopamine	chlorpromazine, etc.
oestrogen receptor	ethinylestradiol	tamoxifen
progesterone receptor	norethisterone	danazol
Ion channel	**Stimulator**	**Blocker**
Na^+ channel in renal tubule	aldosterone	amiloride, triamterene
voltage-gated Ca^{2+} channel in heart and arterioles	no drug	dihydropyridines (e.g. nifedipine, etc.)
ATP-sensitive K^+ channels in pancreatic beta cell		sulphonylureas (e.g. gliclazide, etc.)
GABA-gated Cl^- channels in CNS	benzodiazepines	flumazenil
Enzyme	**Enhancer**	**Inhibitor**
COX-1 and COX-2		NSAIDs, e.g. ibuprofen
ACE		ACE inhibitors, e.g. captopril
HMG-CoA reductase		statins, e.g. simvastatin
dihydrofolate reductase		trimethoprim, methotrexate
DNA synthetases		azathioprine
5 alpha-reductase		finasteride
aromatase		anastrozole, etc.
Carrier	**Accelerator**	**Inhibitor**
noradrenaline reuptake	amphetamines	tricyclic antidepressants
serotonin reuptake		SSRIs
'proton pump' (H^+/K^+-ATPase)		proton pump inhibitors, e.g. omeprazole
cardiac 'Na^+/K^+ pump' (Na^+/K^+-ATPase)		cardiac glycosides, e.g. digoxin
renal tubular ion carriers		all diuretics

excretion of drugs by the renal tubule, which was described in Chapter 4. Among the most commonly prescribed drugs in primary care are several that block carriers.

The proton-pump inhibitors block the H^+/K^+ exchanger in the gastric mucosa (*see* Figure 8.4). Digoxin blocks the Na^+/K^+ pump in cardiac muscle. The loop diuretics block the $Na^+/K^+/2Cl^-$ co-transporter in the loop of Henle. Finally, the tricyclic antidepressants (TCAs) block the carrier mechanism responsible for noradrenaline uptake at the synaptic cleft.

Conclusion

It is hoped that this chapter will have given readers a clear concept of the varied mechanisms by which different prescribed drugs achieve their therapeutic benefit. Table 8.1 shows the four most significant cellular targets of some important drugs prescribed in primary care.

It is worth noting that with every new drug discovery has come a better understanding of molecular biology, which in turn has led to more precise focusing of the search for even better drugs.

Key points

- There are four known targets for drug action.
- A drug may act at either a receptor, an ion channel, an enzyme or a carrier mechanism.
- Drugs acting on enzymes or carrier mechanisms have mostly been discovered in the last 30 years.
- They include drugs to block enzymes involved in inflammation, excess cholesterol, advanced breast cancer and benign prostatic hyperplasia.
- Drugs acting on carrier mechanisms include the diuretics and drugs to treat depression, peptic ulceration and heart disease.
- A table summarises the four drug targets, with examples of each type of drug.

9 Calcium ion for the prescriber

As we have already seen, many of the most important chemicals involved in cell signalling are simple ions such as potassium, sodium, calcium and chloride. Calcium ion is one of the most important of these, modulating cellular metabolism, so its concentration in the cell cytoplasm is very strictly regulated. Box 9.1 gives a list of the main functions of calcium ion.

Box 9.1 The main functions of calcium ion.

- Regulates muscle contraction – smooth, skeletal and cardiac muscle.
- Regulates the release of many neurotransmitters and hormones.
- Regulates/controls permeability of cell membranes to other ions.
- Regulates the activities of many intracellular enzymes.
- Has 'secondary messenger' functions (secondary messengers are intracellular mediators, e.g. between a receptor and an enzyme; *see* Chapter 5).
- Depolarisation of many excitable tissue cells, including most nerve terminals.

Because of the importance in family practice of calcium-channel blockers such as nifedipine, the rest of this chapter will concentrate on item 1 in Box 9.1 – regulation of muscle contraction. Muscles will not contract without calcium ion, whether they be smooth, skeletal or cardiac. Calcium ion does two things in the muscle cell.

1 It activates the sequence which produces the energy for muscle contraction – ATP/ADP, without which there can be no contraction.
2 It activates the cross-bridging between actin and myosin in muscle cells, which is the process by which chemical energy is transformed into mechanical energy.

The reason why we can use calcium-channel blockers to control cardiac dysfunction without affecting skeletal muscle function is that the source of calcium ion for muscle contraction varies between the three muscle types.

1   *Heart muscle* – calcium enters heart muscle from the extracellular fluid in a controlled
    way via voltage-sensitive L, N and T calcium channels (*see* Figure 9.1). This is the so-
    called 'slow calcium current' (*see* Figure 9.2). The L-type channels predominate in the
    myocardium, while the T-type channels occur mainly in the sinu-atrial node (the
    pacemaker), and the conducting tissues of the heart.

2   *Vascular smooth muscle* – calcium ion enters from the extracellular fluid via L and T
    calcium channels and further calcium is recruited from intracellular stores.

3   *Skeletal muscle* – calcium is released from intracellular stores (the sarcoplasmic
    reticulum). Cell membrane calcium ion channels are not involved.

Clearly, calcium-channel blockers will affect heart muscle and vascular smooth muscle, but
not skeletal muscle.

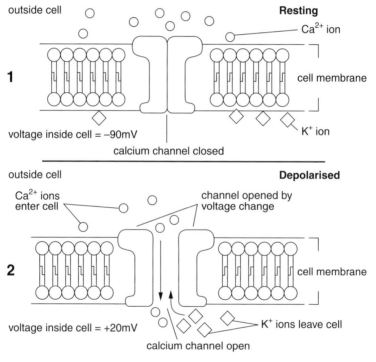

Figure 9.1 The voltage-gated ion channel as a drug target. Calcium enters heart muscle
from the extracellular fluid via the voltage-sensitive L, N, and T calcium channels, which
open in response to depolarisation.

How do calcium-channel blockers work?

When the cell membrane of a cardiac or smooth muscle cell undergoes voltage change
(depolarisation), the voltage-gated calcium ion channels in the membrane open. This allows

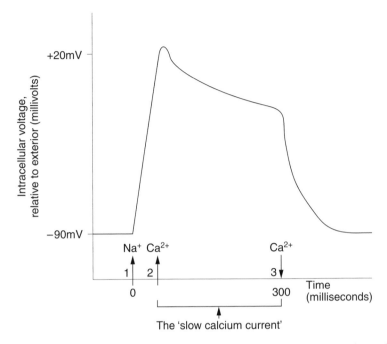

Figure 9.2 The electrical and ionic events of cardiac contraction. (1) Initial rapid depolarisation, caused by opening of voltage-gated Na^+ channels. (2) Slower, prolonged opening of voltage-gated Ca^{2+} channels, resulting in contraction. (3) Repolarisation by extrusion of Ca^{2+} by Ca^{2+} pump mechanisms. (1)–(3) includes the QRST of the classical ECG.

calcium ion to enter the cell from the extracellular fluid, initiating the sequence of contraction. Calcium-channel antagonists, such as nifedipine, bind selectively to these calcium channels in their closed phase, maintaining closure and preventing calcium ion from entering. This reduces the force of contraction, leading to a reduction of cardiac work and increased peripheral arteriolar vasodilation, with a reduction in hypertension.

Why are the nifedipine group (the dihydropyridines) so safe?

As every clinician knows, there are major differences in the uses and safety margins between the three main types of calcium blockers – the nifedipine group, verapamil and diltiazem. The best current explanation for this is that only the L-type channel is sensitive to the nifedipines (the dihydropyridines). Now, L channels predominate in the smooth muscle of the peripheral arterioles, maintaining the appropriate level of arteriolar constriction to maintain blood pressure in normal health. In hypertension, the nifedipine group of

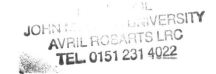

Table 9.1 Choosing the right calcium-channel blocker depends on its predominant site of action.

Drug	Concentration of its recognition sites	Resulting useful therapeutic effects
Nifedipine	Peripheral vascular smooth muscle +++ Coronary smooth muscle ++ Cardiac muscle + Cardiac pacemaker/conductors +	• Strong hypotensive effect • Anti-anginal effect • Weak conduction effect • Weak negative inotropic effect Overall: relatively safe in general practice
Verapamil	Peripheral vascular smooth muscle ++ Coronary smooth muscle ++ Cardiac muscle ++ Cardiac pacemaker/conductors ++	• Good hypotensive effect • Anti-anginal effect • Reduces contractility* • Strong conduction effect** Overall: use with caution in general practice
Diltiazem	Peripheral vasculature + Coronary vasculature ++ Cardiac muscle ++ Pacemaker/conductors +++	• Good hypotensive effect • Good in vasospastic angina • Reduces contractility* • Strong conduction effect** Overall: use with caution in general practice

 * liable to precipitate heart failure
** may worsen conduction defects

calcium-channel blockers cause excellent, sustained peripheral vasodilation by L-calcium-channel blockade in the arteriolar smooth muscle. Cardiac contractility is also reduced somewhat, but the sympathetic baroreceptor reflex is sufficient to maintain cardiac output. Into the bargain, all members of the nifedipine group powerfully dilate the coronary vessels. Hence, we have a very useful therapeutic package, whose main side-effects are a consequence of the primary drug action – flushing and peripheral oedema. Table 9.1 shows the main pharmacological differences between the three groups of calcium-channel blockers, with their relative therapeutic benefits.

Verapamil and diltiazem – use with care!

Why do verapamil and diltiazem depress cardiac contractility and conduction so much more powerfully than the nifedipine group of calcium-channel blockers (*see* Table 9.1)? Currently,

Table 9.2 Therapeutic differences of the dihydropyridines.

Drug	Comment
Nifedipine (the 'bench mark')	Does all that is required, safely, but must be given in sustained-release (SR) form – its short half-life leads to reflex tachycardia between doses
Nicardipine	Equally good, with fewer side-effects. Must also be given in SR form. Decreases the frequency of angina and improves exercise tolerance in exercise-induced angina
Amiodipine	As effective as nifedipine, but its long half-life (>36 hours) reduces the risk of reflex tachycardia
Felodipine	An even better peripheral vasodilator than nifedipine, and has negligible negative inotropic effect on heart muscle
Isradipine	Produces good peripheral vasodilation. Selectively inhibits the cardiac pacemaker (SA node), eliminating reflex tachycardia – the so-called negative chronotropic effect. Has no effect on the general myocardium. Can be used with beta-blockers in appropriate circumstances
Nimodipine	Its high lipid solubility allows it to enter the CNS, hence it is used to relax destructive cerebral vasospasm following subarachnoid haemorrhage

the best theory is that after cardiac contraction, the calcium ion which entered the muscle fibre at the start of contraction must be pumped out again, into both the extracellular fluid (by the Na^+/Ca^{++} pump) and the cardiac intracellular calcium store (by the ATP-dependent calcium pump). Both verapamil and diltiazem delay this recovery process (repolarisation), but members of the nifedipine group do not.

Of major clinical importance, it has recently been found that the effects of both verapamil and diltiazem are enhanced when the heart-rate rises (in exercise or fear), leading to a profound negative inotropic effect and a high risk of precipitating heart failure. This effect is not seen with the nifedipine group of calcium-channel blockers. Thus in primary care, the benefits and safety of this group are obvious. That being so, it is well worth knowing the relative advantages of the different dihydropyridines available to the prescriber: they are by no means identical in action. Table 9.2 summarises the differences and suggests relative indications. In general, the decision to prescribe verapamil or diltiazem should be shared with a consultant cardiologist.

What of the T-calcium ion channels?

As described above, T-calcium channels are present mainly in the cardiac conductive tissue. The pharmaceutical industry is currently searching for a selective calcium T-channel blocker which would have the advantage of reducing the activity of the cardiac pacemaker and protecting the diseased heart from rate increases due to adrenergic stimuli resulting from emotional and other stresses. This should make T-channel blockers particularly useful in hypertensive patients with angina. Mibefradil, the original T-channel blocker, had to be withdrawn because of side-effects, so the search goes on. (It was found that mibefradil inhibited the metabolism of some 30 other drugs (*see* Chapter 3), leading to toxic plasma concentrations of these other drugs. This type of adverse drug interaction is described in Chapter 12.)

Left ventricular hypertrophy and calcium ion

Finally, left ventricular hypertrophy is associated with excess retention of calcium ion within cardiac muscle. Verapamil alone of the older L-calcium-channel blockers is effective in normalising cardiac function in such cases, though ACE inhibitors appear to share this important effect. In addition, verapamil may reduce hypercalcinosis in hypertensive arterial walls. Further, secretion of aldosterone by the adrenal medulla is dependent on T-calcium channels. These are all good reasons for treating moderate-to-severe hypertension with calcium-channel blockers, for left ventricular hypertrophy is present in 20% of all hypertensive patients, greatly worsens their prognosis, and is often missed on ECG. Hypertensive patients with other risk factors such as hyperlipidaemia, obesity and a history of smoking should be referred for echocardiography. Regression of left ventricular hypertrophy can be achieved in its early stages by prompt management of the hypertension which causes it. Otherwise it is largely irreversible.

Key points

- The main functions of calcium ion are listed.
- The chapter then focuses on the role of calcium ion in muscle contraction.
- The voltage-gated calcium ion channel is described.
- Calcium ion is a key feature of cardiac contraction.
- Different calcium-channel blockers have stronger or weaker effects on the different parts of the cardiovascular system.
- Understanding these differences helps the prescriber to select the optimal drug in each patient.
- The enlargement (hypertrophy) of the wall of the left ventricle is associated with excess retention of calcium ion.

10 The scientific basis of prescribing for the elderly

Older people account for a growing percentage of the UK population, and for around one-third of primary care workload and prescribing volume. Unfortunately, several studies in European acute geriatric hospital departments have shown that 10–12% of all acute admissions of elderly patients and 18% of elderly deaths are the direct result of prescribed medicines.[1–3]

Drug:drug interaction is one of the commonest causes of these admissions, along with patient confusion as to the dosage sequence of several concurrent prescriptions. Such confusion may result in an excessively high dose, particularly of psychotropic drugs.

Hyperkalaemia or hyponatraemia is caused by chronic diuretic therapy without proper monitoring of blood electrolytes. Build up of plasma drug concentrations due to reduced liver and kidney function is common. One or more of the well-known side-effects and interactions of NSAIDs, which were considered in Chapter 7, are common causes of drug-associated illness in the elderly.

Box 10.1 A large proportion of all ADRs occur in elderly patients, but these are vastly under-reported.

The problem
Over-65s account for:

- 33% of all prescriptions
- 27% of all reported ADRs; ratio female:male = 2:1
- 15% of population.

The reasons
Over-65s have:

- decreased salivation and swallowing, protein binding, drug metabolism/elimination
- altered drug-tissue distribution and drug-tissue responses
- unavoidable polypharmacy.

Box 10.1 summarises the problem and highlights that 27% of all adverse drug reactions (ADRs) reported to the CSM occur in the elderly; it also gives the underlying reasons for this iatrogenic phenomenon.

The biological age of elderly patients

There is no such thing as a standard prescription for an elderly patient. Therefore it is important to assess the patient's biological age, i.e. are they a 'senior athlete' or are they chronically ill with multiple organ failure and pathology?

Common to all patients over the age of 70 are the physiological changes of ageing, leading to a gradual reduction in functional reserve in the cardiovascular, respiratory, renal, hepatic, musculoskeletal and central nervous systems, as well as the skin.

Whether a patient's presenting symptoms are due to normal physiological ageing, requiring only reassurance, or to pathology requiring drug treatment, is often a difficult clinical judgement.

Reduced drug metabolism and excretion

Tables 10.1–10.3 show the essential therapeutic considerations that every prescriber should check off whenever issuing or repeating a prescription for an older patient. The check-list consists of altered liver and kidney function, nutrition, tissue responses and body composition.

In Chapters 3 and 4 we considered drug metabolism and excretion, and Table 10.1 shows that decreased drug metabolism and excretion are normal in older patients, particularly those over the age of 70.

If standard adult doses of many drugs are given to this age group, excessive plasma concentrations will gradually accumulate. The problem is exacerbated by reduced kidney function and a resulting reduction in the ability to excrete drugs and their metabolites. The plasma half-lives of digoxin, lithium and gentamicin are doubled, while that of diazepam may be quadrupled.

The common prescription of NSAIDs for joint pain frequently accelerates this natural decline in renal function by inhibiting renal prostaglandin synthesis, causing tubular ischaemia and retention of sodium and water, which may precipitate or worsen left ventricular failure.

Poor nutrition

It is clearly impossible for the nurses, pharmacists and family doctors to be aware of the nutritional status of all their elderly patients, but it is essential to run a mental check-list of nutritional changes whenever prescribing for the elderly (*see* Table 10.2).

Table 10.1 The normal ageing process – changes in liver and kidney function.

Liver changes	Kidney changes
decreased blood flow leads to decreased presystemic drug metabolism	the number of nephrons decreases by 6% per decade; although serum creatinine may be normal, older people do have reduced renal function; at 70, renal function is, at best, 50% of its original maximum
decreased liver size, microsomal (P450) oxidation and antipyrine clearances lead to decreased hepatic drug metabolism	decreased glomerular filtration rate and tubular secretion lead to an increased possibility of accumulation of all drugs and metabolites eliminated via the kidneys
	N.B. NSAIDs can accelerate the decline in renal function, particularly in the presence of cardiac failure

Table 10.2 The normal ageing process – changes in nutrition and tissue responses.

Nutrition changes	Tissue response changes
• vitamins decrease • proteins decrease • nicotine intake unchanged • alcohol intake unchanged	• reduction of brain cells increases effects of psychoactive drugs • reduction of baroreceptor activity increases postural hypotensive effect of drugs • exaggerated response to anticoagulants; increased risk of gastrointestinal bleeding with NSAIDs

Table 10.3 The normal ageing process – changes in body composition.

Changes in body composition	Result
• decreased body weight • decreased body water • increased body fat percentage • decreased plasma albumin	• increased effect of standard dose • increased plasma concentration of water-soluble drugs • decreased plasma concentration of fat-soluble drugs • reduced protein binding

The community dietitian should be asked to survey the nutritional status of less healthy elderly patients on chronic medication and be asked about and involved in treatment planning.

Changes in tissue responses and body composition

The elderly have increased tissue sensitivity to several commonly-needed CNS and cardiovascular drug groups, including the opioid analgesics, the antipsychotics, the anti-parkinsonian drugs, the benzodiazepines and digoxin (*see* Table 10.2). The *BNF* clearly indicates which drugs require dosage reduction in the elderly, and some drugs have geriatric formulations, for example digoxin 62.5 μg.

Body composition changes are also important to remember, particularly in patients aged over 75 years, as the reductions in body weight, body water and plasma albumin all conspire to increase the plasma drug concentration and the effect of many medicines (*see* Table 10.3).

Therefore, it is clear that prescribing for the elderly requires a thorough knowledge of the practical pharmacology that this book has attempted to bring to the prescriber.

Suggestions for rational geriatric prescribing

Box 10.2 lists points to consider when prescribing for senior citizens, particularly if you are considering prescribing an hypnotic, diuretic, NSAID, digoxin, antihypertensive, antiparkinsonian, a psychotropic drug or warfarin.

Box 10.2 Points to consider when prescribing for elderly patients.

- What is his or her biological age, i.e. is the patient fit for his or her age or should special care with medication be taken due to overt organ failure?
- Should a low starting dose be used (e.g. calcium-channel blockers, many antidepressants, all benzodiazepines)?
- Has this drug a small margin of safety (e.g. digoxin, theophylline, lithium, warfarin)?
- What is its route of elimination (e.g. avoid chlorpropamide and glibenclamide in any degree of renal impairment)?
- What interactions may occur with the existing treatment?
- Could the new drug worsen existing pathology (e.g. NSAIDs)?

Box 10.3 lists questions for every medication review, which should be conducted at the time of the patient's annual clinical review, or more often, if indicated.

Box 10.3 Questions to consider when reviewing the current long-term drug treatment of elderly patients.

- Is it strictly necessary?
- Is it being taken?
- Are there side-effects?
- Is it having any therapeutic effect?
- Are any of the drugs incompatible?

Box 10.4 Some rules for prescribers when treating the elderly.

- Keep prescribing simple – as few drugs as possible, but polypharmacy may be unavoidable.
- Once- or twice-daily regimens may improve compliance, particularly if associated with mealtimes.
- Encourage a balanced diet – meals on wheels, dietitian, etc.
- Reduce smoking and alcohol intake as much as possible.
- Clear, large labelling is essential.
- Small tablets make swallowing easier.
- Avoid modified-release (SR, LA) products unless they are pharmacologically justified, e.g. the short half-lives of nifedipine and diltiazem make them unsuitable for use except in the SR/LA formulation; note that when prescribing maintenance treatment using any SR/LA formulation, the same brand name should always be used due to variations in pharmacokinetics between brands.
- Avoid fixed-dose combinations, unless they aid compliance.
- Do not use NSAIDs for analgesia only.
- Consider the individual's biological age, not chronological age.

Prescribers should be aware of the common problem of co-morbidity in the elderly, leading to unavoidable polypharmacy. This problem is now compounded for the prescriber by the advent of compelling research-based evidence showing the proven benefits of many drug treatments.

This evidence may indicate that a given patient should be prescribed digoxin, a loop diuretic, an ACE inhibitor, a low-dose cardioselective beta-blocker, warfarin *and* a statin, for example. However, the risk of a serious ADR (*see* Chapters 12 and 13) from such an evidence-based combination is greater than 50%, so the decision to prescribe particular treatments has to be based on experience and knowledge of the patient, as well as research evidence.

Box 10.4 gives suggested general rules for the prescriber when treating elderly patients. Boxes 10.2–10.4 if followed, could improve the health and well-being of your ailing elderly patients, reduce your workload, and greatly reduce the iatrogenic admission rate mentioned at the beginning of this chapter. You may think them worth copying for your practice.

Conclusion

Prescribing for the elderly is probably the most scientifically demanding area of primary care, but the benefits for the patient and the intellectual satisfaction for the prescriber are well worth the effort.

The Royal College of Physicians' report on prescribing for the elderly covers this subject in great detail.[4]

Key points

- 27% of all reported adverse drug events occur in the elderly.
- 10–12% of all acute (emergency) hospital admissions in the over-70s are caused by prescribed drugs.
- The anatomical and physiological changes of ageing (listed in this chapter) are partly responsible for these problems.
- The evidence-based co-prescribing of several drugs to treat degenerative disease is another major factor.
- Confusion and poor compliance often contribute.
- The prescriber must select drugs and adjust dosages to take into account reduced liver and kidney function, body composition changes, deficient nutrition and altered tissue responses in the elderly.
- General guidelines are presented in tabular form.

References

1 Pirmohmed M, Breckenridge AM, Kitteringham NR *et al.* (1998) Adverse drug reactions. *BMJ.* **316**: 1295–8.

2 Williamson J and Chaplin JM (1980) Adverse drug reactions to prescribed drugs in the elderly: a multicentre investigation. *Age and Ageing.* **9**: 73–80.

3 Ebbeson J, Buajordet I, Erikssen J *et al.* (2001) Drug-related deaths in a department of internal medicine. *Arch Intern Med.* **161**: 2317–23.

4 Royal College of Physicians (1997) *Medication for Older People* (2e). Royal College of Physicians, London.

11 Antibacterial action and bacterial resistance

In almost all age groups, antibacterials are the most frequently prescribed drugs in general practice.[1] For five decades, we have had the previously unheard-of power to combat almost all bacterial infections. Unfortunately, this 'antibacterial era' is now under serious threat, and could come to an end within the next 20 years if changes are not made.

Already, patients in hospital are dying of systemic infections resistant to all antibacterials. Moreover, common pathogens, such as *Pneumococcus, Streptococcus pyogenes, Helicobacter pylori* and *Mycobacterium tuberculosis* among others, are showing increasing levels of resistance in the community.

In this chapter, we shall consider the differences in structure and function of the bacterial cell from that of the human host cell, and how these differences are exploited by antibacterials. Then we will deal with the different types of antibacterial resistance, and how these are transferred within and between bacterial populations.

The scientific use of antibacterials depends on a thorough understanding of these principles.

Bacterial and human cells – vive la différence! (see Figure 11.1)

Mammalian cells are much more complex than bacterial cells. The evolutionary proliferation of organelles in human cells has resulted in biochemical functions several orders of magnitude more complex than those of bacteria.

Yet bacterial structure and function are highly refined and have adapted the many thousands of bacterial species to life in every known environment: geological, botanical and zoological, including, of course, the human body. Billions of bacteria live in the human body symbiotically, and occasionally as pathogens.

Antibacterial drugs exploit the differences between bacterial and human cell structure in order to avoid affecting the human host cells, although there are some risks to patients (*see* Figure 11.1 and Table 11.1).

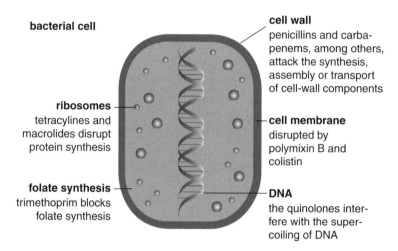

bacterial cell

cell wall
penicillins and carba-
penems, among others,
attack the synthesis,
assembly or transport
of cell-wall components

ribosomes
tetracylines and
macrolides disrupt
protein synthesis

cell membrane
disrupted by
polymixin B and
colistin

folate synthesis
trimethoprim blocks
folate synthesis

DNA
the quinolones inter-
fere with the super-
coiling of DNA

Figure 11.1 Antibacterial targets in the bacterial cell, and examples of the antibacterials that act at these sites (*see* also Table 11.1).

No bacterial nucleus or organelles

The most obvious difference between human and bacterial cells is that the bacterium has no nucleus, mitochondria, Golgi apparatus or endoplasmic reticulum. Instead, it has a single chromosome without a nuclear membrane, which consists of a tightly-wound (supercoiled) DNA molecule lying within the bacterial cytoplasm.

Enzymes control the local uncoiling and recoiling of the chromosome so that biological functions can occur. Some antibacterials, such as ciprofloxacin, block the action of the enzyme topoisomerase II, which is a DNA gyrase (*see* Table 11.1).

The rigid bacterial cell wall

Another major target for antibacterials is the cell wall. Although both human and bacterial cells have a phospholipid cell membrane, almost all bacteria have an additional, relatively rigid, outer cell wall. The function of the cell wall is to support the underlying cell membrane, which is under high osmotic pressure and would otherwise burst.

The key component of the cell wall is a substance called peptidoglycan, which is unique to bacteria, and can therefore be exploited by many antibacterials (*see* Table 11.1). These antibacterials disrupt the synthesis or assembly of cell wall components at various sites, or their transport out of the cell.

The cell wall target becomes more complex, however, when Gram-negative bacteria are taken into consideration. These have an additional outer lipoprotein and lipopolysaccharide membrane, which allows them to exclude a wide variety of antibacterials. By contrast, Gram-positive bacteria do not have an external membrane, and can therefore be more easily

Table 11.1 How and where antibacterials attack bacteria.

Bacterial structure	Antibacterials that attack this target	Mode of action
bacterial cell wall (peptidoglycan)	penicillins, monobactams, carbapenems, cephalosporins and cephamycin	prevent cross-linkage of peptidoglycan, preventing bacterial cell wall completion
	vancomycin, teicoplanin	inhibit addition of bacterial wall components
bacterial cell membrane	polymyxin B and colistin	disrupt bacterial cell membrane via a 'detergent' action
bacterial protein synthesis (via messenger RNA)	tetracyclines, erythromycin and other macrolides, chloramphenicol, neomycin, streptomycin and other aminoglycosides	disrupt a specific step of bacterial protein synthesis
	rifampicin and other rifamycins	inhibit bacterial RNA polymerase, preventing its transcription to code protein synthesis
bacterial chromosome	ciprofloxacin and other quinolones	disrupt supercoiling of the bacterial chromosome by inhibiting DNA gyrase
	trimethoprim, sulphonamides	disrupt folate synthesis, thus preventing DNA synthesis

affected by the antibacterial mechanisms described above. The bacterial cell membrane can also be attacked directly and disrupted by so-called 'detergent antibacterials', such as the polymyxins.

Bacterial protein synthesis

Protein synthesis on messenger RNA templates is different in bacterial and human cells. The tetracyclines, aminoglycosides (e.g. streptomycin), chloramphenicol and the macrolides (e.g.

erythromycin), among others, exploit this difference at one or more of the six steps in the protein-assembly process.

The rifamycins (e.g. rifampicin) and metronidazole interfere with aspects of DNA and RNA function, such as metabolism and reproduction.

The bacterial folate synthesis mechanism

Lastly, the commonly-used folate antagonist, trimethoprim, and the now rarely-used sulphonamides, block the synthesis of folate within the bacterium, prior to its use in DNA synthesis. This action effectively blocks DNA function at its earliest possible stage.

It is clear then that there are several ways in which antibacterials can disrupt bacterial function. Bacteria, however, are able to evolve quickly and can develop resistance to these attacks.

Natural selection – the biological imperative

Bacteria, like all living organisms, undergo occasional mutations, a small proportion of which result in new strains that are more able to resist antibacterial attack. Because of the size of bacterial populations – there are probably more bacteria in the human intestine than there are cells in the human body – and because of their frequency of replication – often once every 20 minutes – the opportunity for developing resistance is enormous. It is unlikely that any antibacterial will be discovered to which bacteria will not develop resistance.

Resistance to antibacterials is promoted by the widespread use of antibacterials and by prolonged courses of treatment. In particular, the unnecessary use of antibacterials for trivial, self-limiting and often viral infections of the upper respiratory tract is a perfect recipe for resistance development. Transfer of resistant bacteria is aided by dirty hospitals, poor infection control techniques, and the close proximity of hospital patients.

The mutant resistant bacteria are often inherently weaker in metabolism than the original 'wild' strains, and cannot establish themselves against the stronger resident bacteria. Therefore, resistant bacteria become a very small fraction of the bacterial flora. However, if an antibacterial is prescribed to a patient, the resistant strain has an enormous advantage: the original bacteria will be eliminated and entirely replaced by a population of the resistant strain.

There is also evidence that natural, commensal bacteria have a role in resisting colonisation by pathogens; for example, commensal *Neisseria* populating the healthy nasopharynx appear to inhibit colonisation by meningococci. This 'colonisation resistance' is an under-recognised defence mechanism. In this and other body areas, e.g. the colon, the use of antibacterials will strip the tissue of its normal, protective flora and facilitate access by pathogens.

How resistance is transferred

Unfortunately, mutations conferring resistance to antibacterials are not restricted to the descendants of the original mutant. The resistance gene can be shared with non-resistant bacteria of the same species and is sometimes transferred to entirely different bacterial species.

This process is known as 'acquired resistance', and is at the core of the problem of antibacterial resistance. It can occur when:

- there is conjugation between bacteria of the same species and strain, which is when resistant genes (DNA) are passed across interconnecting tubules via plasmids. The gene is not incorporated in the bacterial chromosome (*see* Figure 11.2①), but since plasmids self-replicate independently of the bacterial chromosome, resistance genes can be transferred very rapidly by this method
- the resistant gene is incorporated into a neighbouring bacterium's chromosome. In this case, the resistant gene is now permanent and will be transferred to all future generations. This occurs when the resistant gene is transferred across a tubule by a transposon (a section of plasmid DNA), which can insert the resistant gene into the bacterial chromosome. Transposons can carry resistant genes between entirely different bacterial species (*see* Figure 11.2②)
- resistance to many antibacterials, known as 'multi-drug resistance', is transferred between bacteria of the same strain and species or to other bacterial species by multi-cassette

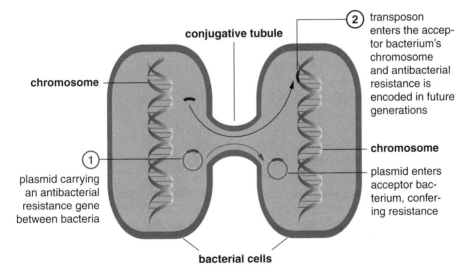

Figure 11.2 Two methods of transfer of antibacterial resistance between bacteria.

arrays of genes resistant to many antibacterials. This is a complex, elegant and probably unique biological process, and examples include the notorious methicillin-resistant *Staphylococcus aureus* (MRSA), which is multi-drug resistant.

The metabolic mechanisms of antibacterial resistance

It remains to describe the biochemical and metabolic processes by which bacteria resist attack by different antibacterials. Once in place, the resistant genes alter the bacterial metabolism in one of five ways, as discussed below (*see* Figure 11.3).[2] Although several hundred different antibacterial resistances have been identified, almost all can be ascribed to one or other of these five classes of resistance.[2]

Enzymatic inactivation (*see* Figure 11.3 ①)

Bacteria can inactivate the antibacterial before it enters the bacterial cell. For example, it is well known that staphylococcal resistance to penicillin is usually due to its ability to produce beta-lactamase, which splits the penicillin molecule.

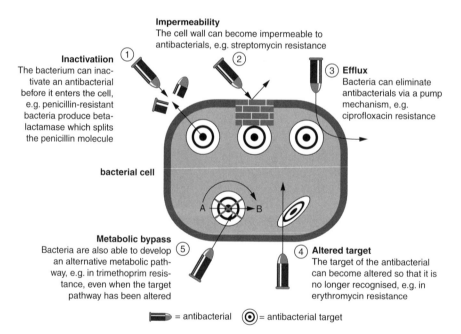

Impermeability
The cell wall can become impermeable to antibacterials, e.g. streptomycin resistance ②

Inactivatiion ①
The bacterium can inactivate an antibacterial before it enters the cell, e.g. penicillin-resistant bacteria produce beta-lactamase which splits the penicillin molecule

③ **Efflux**
Bacteria can eliminate antibacterials via a pump mechanism, e.g. ciprofloxacin resistance

bacterial cell

A → B

Metabolic bypass ⑤
Bacteria are also able to develop an alternative metabolic pathway, e.g. in trimethoprim resistance, even when the target pathway has been altered

④ **Altered target**
The target of the antibacterial can become altered so that it is no longer recognised, e.g. in erythromycin resistance

= antibacterial   ◎ = antibacterial target

Figure 11.3 The five classes of bacterial resistance. From *Resistance to Antibacterials and Other Microbial Agents*,[2] reproduced with permission from the Controller of Her Majesty's Stationery Office.

It is of some interest, following our discussion of enzyme induction in Chapter 3, that the beta-lactamase enzyme is actually induced by the presence of minute amounts of any penicillin or other beta-lactam antibacterial, including the cephalosporins.

Beta-lactamase diffuses from the bacterium, through its cell membrane and cell wall, inactivating the antibacterial molecules in its vicinity.

Cell-wall or membrane impermeability (see Figure 11.3②)

The bacterial cell wall and/or plasma membrane can become impermeable to the antibacterial, making it ineffective. Examples of this are resistance to the aminoglycosides, the beta-lactams, chloramphenicol and the tetracyclines.

Pump mechanism (see Figure 11.3③)

Bacteria can develop a pump mechanism for extruding the antibacterial molecule (efflux). This is a common mechanism of resistance to ciprofloxacin and the other quinolones, as well as the tetracyclines.

Altered target (see Figure 11.3④)

The antibacterial's metabolic 'target', e.g. an enzyme within the bacterium, can become altered so that there is no longer a recognition site for the antibacterial. This is the main mechanism of resistance to erythromycin and the other macrolides.

Bypass mechanism (see Figure 11.3⑤)

Finally, bacteria can develop an alternative metabolic pathway or 'bypass' when the antibacterial has reached and disabled its metabolic target. The classic example is bacterial resistance to trimethoprim, in which resistant bacteria have developed an alternative pathway for folic acid synthesis that is insensitive to trimethoprim.

What can be done to preserve the 'antibacterial era'?

Unfortunately, in the majority of cases, resistance against current antibacterials is already encoded in the bacterial chromosome and is not susceptible to any known measures. As already mentioned, although resistant bacteria are generally biologically weaker than the wild strains, following the prescription of antibacterials they will be able to multiply rapidly and occupy the newly available habitat within a few days.

In order to avoid antibacterials becoming obsolete (*see* Table 11.2), it is generally recommended that antibacterial use by GPs, vets and farmers should be reduced to an

Table 11.2 Examples of valuable antibacterial therapies now lost or imperilled by the spread of resistance.[2]

Organism	Disease	Agents lost or threatened
Pneumococcus	pneumonia, otitis media, meningitis	penicillin; many others
Meningococcus	meningitis, septicaemia	sulphonamides, penicillin
Haemophilus influenzae	meningitis	ampicillin, chloramphenicol
Staphylococcus aureus	wound infection, sepsis	penicillin, penicillinase-resistant penicillins, others
Salmonella typhi	typhoid fever	most relevant agents
Shigella	bacillary dysentery	most relevant agents
Gonococcus	gonorrhoea	sulphonamides, penicillin, tetracycline (ciprofloxacin)
E. coli (coliforms)	urinary infection, septicaemia	ampicillin, trimethoprim, others
multi-drug resistant organisms	many hospital infections	most antibiotics

unavoidable minimum, i.e. when there is evidence of significant, systemic bacterial infection. The narrowest spectrum drug should be used, according to the practitioner's knowledge of local bacterial sensitivities.

Next, hospitals must return to previous stringent hygienic and nursing standards and reintroduce the time-consuming techniques of strict barrier nursing of both infected and vulnerable (non-infected) patients.

Public education must continue in order to change the expectation that antibacterials will be prescribed for minor, self-limiting infections.

Finally, as new antibacterials are developed, regulatory agencies, such as the CSM in the UK, must take stringent measures to ensure that these precious, new and vulnerable resources are restricted in use to hospital patients only, and even then only on the advice of a medical microbiologist.

It is hoped that this chapter has provided a useful understanding of bacteria and antibacterials, which are subjects of great importance in general practice.

Key points

■ Antibacterial drugs exploit four major differences between human and bacterial cells.

■ A given antibacterial disrupts one of these four elements of bacterial structure and function, killing the bacterium without harming the human cells.

■ Bacteria have evolved five distinct metabolic resistance mechanisms to evade antibacterial attack, via mutation of bacterial DNA.

■ A bacterium can transfer its resistance genes to other bacteria of the same species and to bacteria of many other, unrelated species.

■ Genes encoding resistance to many antibacterials have been transferred to many pathogenic bacterial species and are now causing major problems worldwide in managing life-threatening infections.

References

1 Connolly JP and McGavock H (1999) Antibacterial prescribing for respiratory tract infections in general practice. *Pharmacoepidemiol Drug Safe.* **8**: 95–104.

2 House of Lords Select Committee on Science and Technology (1998) *Resistance to Antibacterials and Other Antimicrobial Agents.* **HL81-II**: 9. HMSO, London.

12 How to prevent adverse drug interactions – ADIs

This chapter is concerned with our using pharmacological knowledge to become safer prescribers. Safer prescribing involves reducing the incidence of prescription-related acute hospital admissions and deaths, not to mention the unnecessary symptoms and morbidity caused by adverse drug interactions (ADIs). Whenever two or more drugs are prescribed for a patient, the prescriber should always consider whether one drug is known to interact with the other(s) in an adverse (harmful) manner, for that is a very common occurrence.

ADIs can usefully be divided into six categories. Table 12.1 gives examples of each of these categories:

1   interactions occurring during drug absorption
2   interactions occurring during drug distribution
3   interactions between drugs at their site of action
4   additive and antagonistic effects of two drugs
5   interactions occurring during drug metabolism
6   interactions due to mismatching of two drugs' plasma half-lives.

It may be useful to consult Appendix 1 of the *BNF* when reading this chapter, for a plethora of examples will be found in each category.

Interactions occurring during drug absorption

Patients should usually be warned not to take antacids containing aluminium, magnesium or calcium just before or at the same time as other drugs because they may impair absorption. Antacids may also breach enteric coatings that may have been added to prevent inactivation of a drug by stomach acid. *BNF*, Appendix 1 advises that absorption of the following drugs, among others, is reduced in the presence of antacid:

- ACE inhibitors and angiotensin-II antagonists
- many commonly-used antibiotics, including azithromycin, ciprofloxacin, most tetracyclines, isoniazid and rifampicin
- the antiepileptics gabapentin and phenytoin

- the antifungals itraconazole and ketoconazole
- the antihistamine fexofenadine, several antimalarials, the phenothiazine antipsychotics, and sulpiride
- the antiviral zalcitabine
- the bisphosphonates
- digoxin
- oral iron
- lansoprazole.

Table 12.1 The main mechanisms of adverse drug interactions.

Phase of drug activity	Mechanisms leading to ADIs	Well-known examples
1 drug absorption	impairment of absorption, leading to therapeutic failure	antacids reduce the absorption of 14 commonly-used drugs/ groups – see text
2 drug distribution	one drug may displace a second drug from its protein binding	verapamil displaces digoxin
3 at receptors or other sites of action	competition for receptor binding	beta-blockers diminish the effect of the antiasthmatic beta$_2$ agonists
4 additive and antagonistic effects of two drugs	additive effects	ACE inhibitors and NSAIDs both reduce aldosterone secretion and in combination may cause dangerous hyperkalaemia
5 metabolism	inhibition or induction of cytochrome P450 enzymes	see text for: 11 important ADIs due to enzyme inhibition and 6 due to enzyme induction
6 mismatching of plasma half-lives when 2 drugs are used simultaneously	rapid excretion of one drug may expose the patient to the adverse effects of the other	failure to give repeated doses of naloxone when treating comatose heroin addicts

These are all true drug:drug interactions occurring before either drug has been absorbed. A similar type of reaction occurs if warfarin or digoxin is taken simultaneously with colestyramine, which prevents their absorption.

Finally, drugs that slow gastric emptying will reduce the rate of absorption of most orally administered drugs. The commonest examples of this in practice are the opiate analgesics. Conversely, drugs such as metoclopramide, which speed gastric emptying, will increase the rate of absorption of most drugs.

Interactions occurring during drug distribution

Many drugs are loosely bound to plasma and tissue proteins during distribution to their effector sites. Where two drugs compete for the same protein-binding sites, one may displace the other from its protein binding, releasing it as active free drug in the plasma. This is usually a transient process of no therapeutic significance; however, verapamil or amiodarone cause displacement of digoxin from protein-binding sites leading to digoxin toxicity.

Likewise, giving aspirin or valproate to a patient stabilised on phenytoin increases the free phenytoin concentration, which may cause short-term toxicity, although this is soon corrected by excretion.

Interactions between two drugs at the site of action

Where two drugs compete for binding sites at the same receptor, ion channel, enzyme or carrier mechanism, a reaction may occur.

The classic example is that cardioselective beta-blockers despite their selectivity for $beta_1$ receptors, which predominate in the heart, still bind to a proportion of $beta_2$ adrenergic receptors in the lungs. This may not only precipitate asthma, but also block the binding of $beta_2$ agonists, such as salbutamol, used in managing an acute asthmatic attack. However, such reactions are avoidable, since they can be predicted from knowledge of the drugs' actions.

Additive and antagonistic effects of two drugs

Drugs with different pharmacological actions but similar therapeutic effects are often used together because of their additive effect. A good example is in the treatment of refractory hypertension, where modern guidelines recommend the use of moderate doses of two or more different antihypertensives rather than a maximum dose of a single drug.

The additive effect is also used in the drug treatment of many cancers and of rheumatoid arthritis.

However, additive effects can also be dangerous, as in the use of ACE inhibitors and NSAIDs, where both drugs reduce aldosterone secretion and in combination may cause dangerous hyperkalaemia. Moreover, drugs that are mildly sedative on their own may cause significant sedation when combined. By the same token some drugs also cancel another drug's effects, for example NSAIDs reduce the efficacy of all antihypertensives, an example of antagonism.

Drug interactions occurring during drug metabolism

The majority of drugs are metabolised in the liver by the bank of isoenzymes collectively known as the cytochrome P450 oxidases (CYP), which usually render the drug inactive or less active and prepare it for renal excretion. Unfortunately, a number of important drugs slow down (inhibit) or speed up (induce) one or more of the CYP enzymatic cycles.

Clearly, inhibition of metabolic enzymes will reduce the rate of elimination of the drugs that those enzymes process, and lead to their build-up in the plasma. Enzyme inducers, conversely, will speed up the elimination of the relevant drugs, leading to therapeutic failure. This is an important cause of serious adverse drug reactions and interactions, which may lead to emergency hospital admissions.

For this reason, we reproduce from Chapter 3 the summary tables of the 11 important enzyme inhibitors and the six important enzyme inducers (*see* Tables 12.2 and 12.3). It would do no harm to keep these as an aide-mémoire to be consulted whenever co-prescribing any drug to a patient who is receiving one of the drugs in the left-hand column of either table.

As always, the *BNF*, Appendix 1 is the definitive source of information on drug interactions.

Interactions due to mismatching of two drugs' plasma half-lives

When two drugs are used together or a drug is used to treat the adverse effects of another drug, it is important to bear in mind the drugs' half-lives.

The classic example, not uncommon in present-day emergency care in the community, is the use of naloxone to treat the stuporous or comatose heroin addict. Naloxone displaces morphine and heroin from opioid mu receptors, and very rapidly reverses opioid toxicity, relieving respiratory depression, hypotension, convulsions and sedation, within minutes.

Unfortunately, the half-life of naloxone is only half to one hour, whereas that of heroin is three to four hours. Thus as soon as the naloxone has been metabolised and excreted, the circulating heroin reoccupies the opioid receptors and the dangerous adverse effects recur. That is why it is essential for a prescriber to have several ampoules of naloxone in his or her emergency bag, as it must be repeated according to clinical need.

A further example of mismatching half-lives is the combined use of a thiazide diuretic with amiloride. The two act logically and synergistically in managing mild hypertension, but are strongly associated with the occurrence of fatal hyponatraemia in elderly patients. The reason for this is that amiloride conserves potassium, but increases sodium excretion in the kidneys, with a half-life of 20 hours. This effect is reversed by the thiazide, but the thiazide half-life is only 2.5 hours. Therefore for the remaining 17.5 hours of the daily combined dose there is a relative unchallenged sodium loss, which over months can result in profound sodium depletion, collapse, emergency admission, and often death.

If such combinations are used, it is essential to carry out regular plasma electrolyte estimations.

Table 12.2 Metabolic enzyme inhibitors: these *increase the effect* of drugs whose metabolism is inhibited.

Enzyme inhibitor	Drugs affected
imidazole anti-fungals, e.g. fluconazole, itraconazole, etc.	acenocoumarol (nicoumalone), alfentanil, antivirals, ciclosporin, corticosteroids, digoxin, felodipine, midazolam, phenytoin, quinidine, rifabutin, sildenafil, sulphonylureas, tacrolimus, theophylline, warfarin
cimetidine	<ul><li>anthelmintics</li><li>antiarrythmics: amiodarone, flecainide, lidocaine (lignocaine), procainamide, propafenone, quinidine</li><li>antibacterials: erythromycin, metronidazole</li><li>anticoagulants: acenocoumarol, warfarin</li><li>antidepressants: amitriptyline, doxepin, moclobemide, nortriptyline</li><li>antiepileptics: carbamazepine, phenytoin, valproate</li><li>antifungals: terbinafine</li><li>antihistamines: loratadine</li><li>antimalarials: chloroquine, quinine</li><li>anxiolytics and hypnotics: benzodiazepines, clomethiazole</li><li>beta-blockers: labetalol, propranolol</li><li>calcium-channel blockers: some</li><li>cytotoxics: fluorouracil</li><li>immunosuppressant: ciclosporin (possibly)</li><li>NSAIDs: azapropazone (possibly)</li><li>opioid analgesics: pethidine</li><li>theophylline</li></ul>
omeprazole	diazepam, digoxin (possibly)
allopurinol	ciclosporin
erythromycin and other macrolides	alfentanil, amiodarone, bromocriptine, cabergoline, carbamazepine, ciclosporin, clozapine, disopyramide, felodipine, midazolam, rifabutin, sildenafil, terfenadine, theophylline, zopiclone
ciprofloxacin	theophylline
sulphonamides	phenytoin
amiodarone	acenocoumarol, ciclosporin, digoxin, flecainide, phenytoin, procainamide, quinidine, warfarin
metronidazole	phenytoin, fluorouracil
SSRIs	benzodiazepines (some), carbamazepine, clozapine, flecainide, haloperidol, phenytoin, propranolol, theophylline, tricyclic antidepressants
calcium-channel blockers – verapamil, diltiazem	alcohol, ciclosporin, digoxin, imipramine, midazolam, nifedipine, phenytoin, quinidine, theophylline

Table 12.3 Metabolic enzyme inducers: these *reduce the effect* of drugs whose metabolism is accelerated.

Enzyme inducer	Drugs affected
barbiturates and primidone*	acenocoumarol (nicoumalone), chloramphenicol, ciclosporin, corticosteroids, digitoxin, disopyramide, doxycycline, gestrinone, indinavir, lamotrigine, levothyroxine (thyroxine), metronidazole, mianserin, oral contraceptives, quinidine, theophylline, tibolone, toremifene, tricyclics, warfarin
phenytoin*	acenocoumarol, ciclosporin, clozapine, corticosteroids, digitoxin, disopyramide, indinavir, itraconazole, ketoconazole, lamotrigine, methadone, mexiletine, mianserin, oral contraceptives, paroxetine, quetiapine, quinidine, theophylline, thyroxine, warfarin
carbamazepine	acenocoumarol, antiepileptics, ciclosporin, corticosteroids, digitoxin, gestrinone, haloperidol, indinavir, mianserin, olanzapine, oral contraceptives, risperidone, theophylline, tibolone, toremifene, tricyclic antidepressants, warfarin
rifamycins	acenocoumarol, atovaquone, benzodiazepines, bisoprolol, carbamazepine, chloramphenicol, chlorpropamide, ciclosporin, cimetidine, corticosteroids, dapsone, digitoxin, diltiazem, disopyramide, fluconazole, fluvastatin, haloperidol, indinavir, itraconazole, ketoconazole, levothyroxine, methadone, mexiletine, nifedipine, oral contraceptives, phenytoin, propafenone, propranolol, quinidine, tacrolimus, terbinafine, theophylline, tolbutamide, tricyclic antidepressants, verapamil, warfarin
griseofulvin	acenocoumarol, ciclosporin, oral contraceptives, warfarin
alcohol	paracetamol (toxic metabolites increased), tolbutamide

Conclusion

It is hoped that by using the information from this chapter, prescribers will be able to avoid some ADIs. Information technology is also useful in this area, as it can be used to screen maintenance regimens for interactions, as well as giving the prescriber warnings when he or she is completing a prescription. Finally, the pharmacist should always be involved in reviewing long-term medication, dosage adjustment and compliance.

The next chapter is concerned with avoiding and dealing with adverse drug reactions due to single drugs.

Key points

■ Adverse drug interactions (ADIs) occur when one drug disrupts the absorption, distribution, action or metabolism of a second drug in a manner harmful to the patient.

■ There are six distinct pharmacological categories of ADI.

■ The mechanisms of these are described and examples given.

■ The most serious ADIs are due to induction or inhibition of metabolic enzymes by one drug, causing inadequate or excessive plasma concentrations, respectively, of a second drug.

■ A practice aide-mémoire is provided.

---

13 How to predict and avoid adverse drug reactions to single drugs – ADRs

In the previous chapter, the different types of adverse drug interaction (ADI) were explored with special reference to their avoidance by GP prescribers. In this chapter, the subject is adverse drug reactions (ADRs) to individual drugs.

Prescribers should be aware that several international classifications of ADRs have been produced for the purposes of epidemiological research and/or drug licensing regulations. These are by no means prescriber-friendly, and this chapter aims to help and inform the reader wishing to reduce the risks of ADRs in his or her patients. The topic will be covered in three sections:

1 Common, predictable ADRs, i.e. ADRs due to the pharmacological or physiological actions of a drug.
2 Rare, unpredictable ADRs, i.e. unavoidable, idiosyncratic ADRs with no obvious link to pharmacology or physiology.
3 ADRs due to inappropriate prescribing.

Common, predictable ADRs

If a particular drug is prescribed, there is a likelihood of one or more predictable ADRs occurring. As explained in previous chapters, drugs that block or stimulate receptors, ion channels, cellular enzymes or cell-membrane carrier molecules will bind to and affect the function not only of the diseased (target) system, but of every binding site in the body for that drug molecule (*see* Table 13.1).

The result of this unwanted stimulation or blockade at non-target sites is an ADR disrupting the normal physiological regulation of one or many body processes. (Even so-called 'selective' drugs produce such disruption, but usually to a lesser extent than non-selective drugs.) Well known examples are the tricyclic antidepressants, the SSRIs, and levodopa.

The individual patient's experience of such side-effects and tolerance of them varies greatly, as do patient reactions to different members of the same therapeutic drug class. That

Table 13.1 Some predictable ADRs and their pharmacological basis.

Drug(s)	ADR	Pharmacological cause
antibiotics	diarrhoea, *Clostridium difficile* colitis, thrush	disruption of normal intestinal flora
beta-blockers	asthma cold extremities heart failure (in standard doses) fatigue (TATT – tired all the time)	bronchoconstriction peripheral vasoconstriction negative inotropic action
calcium-channel blockers	headache, peripheral oedema, flushing, palpitations, heart block (diltiazem and verapamil only)	peripheral vasodilatation, blocking of cardiac conducting system
digoxin	arrhythmias, heart block	slowing of AV conduction
immunosuppressants	susceptibility to infection, increased risk of cancers	depression of immune system
levodopa	hypomania, psychosis, nausea, vomiting	action on many cerebral dopaminergic neurones
loop diuretics	hypokalaemia, hyponatraemia, hypomagnesaemia, increased calcium excretion, hypotension	diuretic activity (on renal tubules)
NSAIDs	peptic ulcer, acute renal failure, exacerbation of asthma	blockade of physiological prostaglandin synthesis
tricyclic antidepressants	drowsiness, dry mouth, blurred vision, constipation, urinary retention, cardiac arrhythmias	disruption of autonomic control (antimuscarinic effect)

is why some patients tolerate a particular NSAID, SSRI or oral contraceptive better, and why it is worth trying different analogues to find the preparation that suits an individual best for long-term treatment. However, it is important to remember that these ADRs are predictable and dose related. Table 13.1 gives some well known examples.

Prostaglandins

A good example of the problems associated with 'blanket' blocking of physiological regulators is the adverse effects due to inhibition of prostanoid production by NSAIDs.

Prostanoids have a variety of physiological actions, including mediation of inflammatory response, renal regulation, vasodilatation, inhibition of gastric acid secretion, increased gastric mucus secretion, and bronchodilatation.

By blocking prostanoid production, NSAIDs can have a range of adverse effects, including peptic ulceration, renal failure, and exacerbation of asthma, in addition to their beneficial effects on inflammation.

Serotonin

The same problem arises with drugs that affect important neurotransmitters. Serotonin, like the prostaglandins, has widespread physiological regulatory functions in the gastrointestinal tract, the smooth muscle of the uterus and bronchial tree, the large and small blood vessels (with paradoxical effects), the platelets, the peripheral nerve endings and, of course, the CNS.

Study of the *BNF* monograph on selective serotonin re-uptake inhibitors (SSRIs) indicates that ADRs include nausea, dyspepsia, abdominal pain, diarrhoea, constipation, nervousness, anxiety, headache, insomnia, convulsions, sweating, hypomania, etc.[1] Here again, there is great individual variation in susceptibility to and tolerance of any of these ADRs.

Where a patient experiences an unacceptable ADR, reduction of dosage will often bring relief, but may also reduce the plasma concentration of the drug to sub-therapeutic levels. In such a case, it is always worth trying a different chemical compound in the same pharmacological class.

Advance warning

All prescribers should be aware of the value of discreetly warning patients in advance that they may experience some side-effects, inviting them to report such side-effects promptly, and having a discussion about them. In many cases, such as the well-known adverse effects of HRT – nausea, breast tenderness, weight gain, fluid retention and headaches – perseverance with the treatment for a few weeks or months will see the physiological readjustment of the body to the drug (often with up- or down-regulation of receptors) and a gradual disappearance of the ADR.

Patients also need to be informed that all drugs have adverse reactions and risks and that there is a trade-off between high probability of benefit and low probability of risk with every prescription, including vaccination.

Cessation of treatment

Finally, all prescribers should be aware of the occurrence of adverse reactions on cessation of treatment. This is usually due to the body's compensatory up- or down-regulation of receptors in response to the drug treatment, leading to a 'rebound phenomenon' when treatment ends.

It is common practice to withdraw many drugs gradually, e.g. antipsychotics, anti-depressants, opiate analgesia and some antihypertensives. Non-compliant patients are particularly prone to this type of ADR. The *BNF* gives clear advice on the withdrawal of these medicines, and the pharmacist must label them accordingly.

Rare, unpredictable ADRs

Rare, unpredictable ADRs are sometimes known as 'idiosyncratic, Type B reactions'. They are fortunately rare (often as infrequent as 1 per 100 000 treatment years) and they cannot be predicted from a drug's known pharmacology.

This means that the postmarketing surveillance of each new medicine depends on the vigilance and spontaneous reporting by doctors, nurses and pharmacists of suspected ADRs via the Department of Health Yellow Card system and the Prescription Event Monitoring scheme run by the Drug Safety Research Unit, Southampton. Type B reactions are often devastating and irreversible and have led to the abandonment of many otherwise useful drugs like thalidomide, practolol, cerivastatin, troglitazone and grepafloxacin. Tear-out yellow cards can be found at the back of every *BNF*. Use them on suspicion – do not await certainty of causality.

Pre-existing susceptibility

In all of these cases, there is evidence that a tiny proportion of patients have a genetic, metabolic or physiological susceptibility to the ADR. This certainly applies to the anaphylactic shock caused by penicillin, streptomycin and vaccines in a small proportion of susceptible patients. It also applies to the occurrence of agranulocytosis due to clozapine, carbimazole and chloramphenicol, and the Stevens-Johnson syndrome (major erythema multiforme) due to NSAIDs, phenytoin and sulphonamides.

Incidence of rare ADRs

Many rare ADRs are immunological in origin. Their rarity is worth emphasising: you might encounter one of these reactions twice in your career. However, on a national basis, such reactions account for the death of several hundred patients annually in the UK.

The only known response to this risk is the high index of suspicion that characterises the experienced prescriber, instant checking with your regional medicines information service as to the possibility of a causal relationship between the drug and the suspected ADR, and immediate withdrawal of the drug. The sooner such a drug is withdrawn, the more likely the patient's survival.

Unpredictable reactions are not dose-related, and may recur after even a minute dosage. Patients should carry a MedicAlert warning if they have experienced such a reaction in the past, e.g. a survivor of Stevens-Johnson syndrome should carry a warning to avoid the causal agent.

Avoiding ADRs: inappropriate prescribing

A large number of ADRs are entirely avoidable. Safe and effective prescribing is dependent on accurate diagnosis, and in general practice this is not always possible. Indeed one of the many skills of general practice is an ability to manage uncertainty, based on an assessment of improbability as much as one of probability.

In such circumstances, drugs are sometimes used inappropriately, the commonest example being the prescription of antibiotics for self-limiting infections of the upper respiratory tract in both sexes and all ages. Where the infection is due to a virus (70% of all upper and lower respiratory infections) the patient is exposed to 100% risk with 0% benefit.

Contraindications

Classic examples of inappropriate prescribing are the use of drugs in patients whose diagnosis contraindicates their use. Research in both the USA and the UK has shown that inappropriate drug use may account for as much as 2.5% of all prescribing. A common example is the use of drugs known to precipitate asthma in a patient with a past history of bronchial asthma. Another frequent example is the prescription of any benzodiazepine to a patient with a diagnosis of depression, since all benzodiazepines worsen depressive symptoms.

NSAIDs will cause deterioration in patients with either heart or renal failure. Heart failure and cardiac conduction problems will be exacerbated by prescribing either of the calcium-channel blockers verapamil or diltiazem. For the past 15 years in the USA, the Medicaid service has screened every GP's prescribing monthly, seeking the many examples of inappropriate prescribing, notifying the doctors involved, and preventing potential future harm to patients.

Conclusion

Chapters 12 and 13 have shown that a proportion of ADIs and ADRs are avoidable using the information that this book has tried to convey. It is unlikely that ADRs will ever be completely eliminated, despite the best efforts of the pharmaceutical industry to produce ever more selective and tolerable drugs and the best efforts of clinicians to make their prescribing an applied science, as it is at its best.

Nevertheless, there is no reason why the incidence of serious, life-threatening ADRs and ADIs should not be greatly reduced using pharmacological knowledge. This can be aided by the regular use of information technology to screen for drug interaction, and by involving community pharmacists more directly in long-term patient care, with therapeutic reviews of medication, searches for side-effects and fostering compliance.

The regional or district Medicines Information Service is an excellent source of help when the prescriber is in doubt regarding any medication; the telephone numbers are listed on the inside front cover of the *BNF*.

In summary, use your pharmacological knowledge to avoid ADRs at the moment of writing the prescription. Then be proactive in seeking out ADRs in your patients, especially the elderly. Respond quickly and appropriately whenever you suspect them. There is no more important or rewarding area of clinical practice.

Key points

■ ADRs can be divided into two categories: predictable and unpredictable.

■ Predictable ADRs are usually dose related and due to the known pharmacology of the drug.

■ Some drugs, such as tricyclic antidepressants, cause side-effects due to their action on receptors in organs other than the target.

■ Patients should be warned in advance of well-known adverse reactions, e.g. from HRT, and urged to persevere.

■ Cessation of treatment can bring about adverse reactions, hence the necessity to withdraw some drugs gradually, e.g. opiates.

■ Unpredictable ADRs are very rare, and can be assigned in some cases to a pre-existing susceptibility in the patient.

■ Drugs such as antibiotics are commonly prescribed inappropriately for self-limiting infections, subjecting patients to risk without benefit.

■ ADRs can occur when drugs are prescribed to patients in whom they are contraindicated.

■ Screening technology, co-operation of the community pharmacist and vigilance can all help to avoid ADRs.

Reference

1 *BNF*, Section 4.3.3. Introductory monograph: Selective serotonin re-uptake inhibitors. Revised twice yearly. BMA/RPSGB, London.

Further reading

• *British National Formulary* (*BNF*), published in March and September each year. BMA/RPSGB, London.

• Hardman JG and Limbird L (2001) *Goodman and Gilman's The Pharmacological Basis of Therapeutics* (10e). McGraw-Hill Education, New York.

• Rang HP, Dale MM and Ritter JM (1999) *Pharmacology* (4e). Churchill Livingstone, Edinburgh.

14 Getting new drugs to market: licensing medicines for human use

If pharmacology is important for the prescriber, it is even more important during the production, testing and licensing of a new drug. Almost the full range of pharmacological knowledge comes into play during this complex process, which can take up to 12 years and cost up to £500 million. The pharmaceutical manufacturer is responsible for all of this preliminary scientific work, at the end of which the company submits a dossier, often running to hundreds of pages in length, to the national drug licensing organisation, e.g. the Medicines Control Agency in the UK and the Food and Drugs Administration in the USA.*
A typical application comprises the following sections:

1 Description of the active chemical compound.
2 Description of the quality control processes during its manufacture.
3 Description of the pharmaceutics – the vehicle (e.g. a powder) in which the active substance is carried, the process of tabletting or preparation of capsules or injectate, etc. Excipients may include additives necessary to stabilise the active chemical compound and, in the case of some injections, antiseptic agents to inhibit the growth of micro-organisms.
4 Description of the mandatory preclinical tests conducted in animal models.
5 Description of the clinical trials carried out in human volunteers and patients, of which there are three phases prior to the licensing and marketing of a new drug.

Preclinical testing

The preclinical phase of drug development involves the testing of the new drug in animal models. This is first to determine its action on the likely human target organ and its additional effects on other organs (the pharmacodynamics). Second, there are extensive tests for toxicity on all the major organ systems, again carried out on suitable animal models. Third, there is the very important and rigorous testing for teratogenicity – the potential to produce cancers. Only after a new drug has cleared all of the research and preclinical hurdles can it be considered for testing in human subjects (see Box 14.1).

---

* Every developed country has its own version of the MCA and FDA.

Box 14.1 The development of new drugs.

Research
Discovery of a new active chemical compound
↓
Preclinical testing
In vitro and animal studies, defining pharmacology and toxicology
↓
Clinical trials (human studies)
↓
Phase 1
Volunteer studies (up to 100 healthy people)
Investigating safety, pharmacokinetics and metabolic effects
↓
Phase 2
Controlled studies in a homogeneous group of patients
(up to 500 patients)
Proving safety, efficacy and dosage range
↓
Phase 3
Testing safety and efficacy in a more heterogeneous population
Pivotal clinical trials (up to 3000 patients)
↓
Submission of dossier to licensing authority
↓
Phase 4
Post-marketing surveillance:

- Ongoing investigation of safety and adverse effects
- Establishing efficacy in the general population
- Determining cost-effectiveness
- Seeking unexpected therapeutic benefits (leading to extension of licence)

Clinical trials: testing a new drug on healthy and sick people

Box 14.1 shows that the clinical trials of a drug are usually grouped in four phases. This is the most critical and risky part of new drug development. The potential of a promising new therapeutic substance to cause harm is a major risk, both to healthy volunteers and to patients with the target disease. As described in previous chapters, drugs are rarely entirely selective for their target receptor, ion channel, enzyme or carrier mechanism, and will affect all similar binding sites, often causing unacceptable side-effects. In addition, there is always the possibility of idiosyncratic adverse reactions, as described in Chapter 13. So volunteers taking part in phases 1, 2 or 3 of clinical trials are monitored with the utmost care and in the greatest possible detail. All research in phases 1–3 must have independent ethical approval before it can proceed.

Phase 1

In phase 1 of the clinical trials, up to 100 healthy volunteers are given the new drug and subjected to physiological, pharmacological and biochemical tests aimed to reveal safety, side-effects, metabolic effects and particularly, the pharmacokinetics of the drug as described in Chapters 1–4 of this book. Such volunteer subjects are carefully screened for pre-test normality. In particular, anyone taking any drug or consuming large amounts of alcohol is excluded, as are any volunteers with any form of detectable biochemical or endocrine abnormality. Subjects are normally paid for their time and in recognition of the risk involved. This phase 1 testing is often done in university departments of pharmacology, or by specialised companies who undertake this work for the product owner.

Phase 2

In phase 2 trials, the new drug is used for the first time in patients suffering from the condition which the drug is expected to benefit, either by rebalancing the disturbed physiology, or by killing cancerous cells or invading micro-organisms. Phase 2 trials are carried out on relatively small numbers – a maximum of 500 patients in most cases – and are usually in the form of randomised, double-blind, controlled clinical trials, in which half of the group receive the new drug while the other half continue to receive their existing treatment or a placebo. Such studies are designed to prove efficacy, to look at safety once again, and to determine the dosage range most likely to be required. Phase 2 studies are unlikely to be predictive of the drug's effects in the general population, because of the exclusions imposed by the overriding need for avoidance of harm. Phase 2 studies, and pre-licensing drug trials generally, exclude the old, children, pregnant women, people taking other drugs, heavy drinkers and smokers, and all drug abusers. So these trials are not conducted on typical primary care patients!

Phase 3

In phase 3 trials, up to 3000 patients with an appropriate diagnosis receive the new drug, usually in the setting of a randomised, blinded, controlled trial lasting anything from three months to a year. From the licensing point of view, phase 3 trials are the most critical, since they are carried out on a relatively heterogeneous population, though with the same exclusions referred to above, and usually in the relatively controlled environment of hospital medicine.

Application to the licensing authority

Following phase 3 clinical trials of a new drug, the parent pharmaceutical company prepares a detailed and very lengthy dossier, reporting all the known facts about the new drug in its possession, to the licensing authority. The various sections of this lengthy file are scrutinised by authority experts in each of the relevant fields: pharmaceutical, toxicological, preclinical and clinical, including a rigorous assessment of the statistical procedures that the company has followed in its trials. The licensing authority may grant authorisation, require the company to conduct further proving tests and resubmit its application, or reject the application. In Europe, this process can now be undertaken in a number of ways. First, on a national basis, which involves licensing the drug for a particular country. Second, the company may opt for a centralised procedure, licensing the drug for the entire European Union. Alternatively, a mutual recognition procedure may be followed, in which authorisation by one member state is followed by submission to the other member states, who may or may not approve the new compound.

Phase 4: post-marketing surveillance

Post-marketing surveillance is in every respect as important as phases 1, 2 and 3, and is often a great deal more difficult to conduct. Once a drug is marketed and widely prescribed by clinicians, who may not always have an adequate understanding of its properties (relying on the advice of consultant colleagues or indeed, of drug industry representatives, for their information) the potential for harm begins to emerge. Added to this is the fact that family doctors are not always as aware of the need for clinical suspicion of adverse events as they might be. It is in phase 4 that the types and incidence of adverse drug reaction and adverse drug interaction are usually defined, a process which may take several years and which may lead to the withdrawal of the drug within a few years of its licensing. On the other hand, post-marketing surveillance may reveal unexpected benefits from a new drug, giving that drug company a marketing advantage. Box 14.1 summarises this long and costly process. Clinical opinion tends to pass through an initial phase of optimism regarding newly licensed drugs – the wonder-drug scenario! If serious adverse effects are revealed, this is often followed by an equally uncritical period of professional distrust, sometimes quite unjustified, as the adverse effects are often related to incorrect use of the new drug. Unfortunately, such distrust may reach a national level, and occasionally result in the withdrawal of a promising new treatment, which if selectively and scientifically used, should have remained available, at least on a consultant-advised basis.

The final phase in a new drug's development is the acceptance phase, in which its known benefits are balanced against its known risks, and its position in the therapeutic armamentarium is accepted worldwide.

Box 14.2 The golden age of drug innovation, 1960–2002.

- Penicillin esters
- Loop diuretics
- Antipsychotics
- Tricyclic antidepressants
- Benzodiazepines
- Cephalosporins
- 4-Quinolones
- Macrolides
- Oral contraceptives
- Hormone replacement therapy
- Beta-blockers
- NSAIDs
- Beta$_2$-adrenoceptor agonists
- Inhaled steroids
- Histamine H$_2$ receptor blockers

- Synthetic prostaglandin analogues
- Calcium-channel blockers
- ACE inhibitors
- Selective serotonin reuptake inhibitors
- Cancer chemotherapy – many powerful agents
- Lipid-lowering agents
- Proton pump inhibitors
- Anti-oestrogens and hypothalamic and pituitary hormones
- New hypoglycaemics
- Antiandrogens
- Monoclonal antibodies
- Antiviral agents

There are perhaps two lessons for the prescriber resulting from the above account. First, to respect the enterprise and effort of the drug industry which has, over the past 40 years, given us a golden age of drug discovery (*see* Box 14.2). Second, to remember that a new drug should rarely be prescribed in the community without the recommendation of a consultant, and that when it is prescribed, the prescriber is responsible for maintaining a high index of suspicion, and reporting on suspicion alone, any perceived adverse effects to the National Pharmacovigilance Authority.

Index